INTERVENING WITH ASSAULTED WOMEN:
CURRENT THEORY, RESEARCH, AND PRACTICE

INTERVENING WITH ASSAULTED WOMEN:
CURRENT THEORY, RESEARCH, AND PRACTICE

Edited by
Barbara Pressman
Gary Cameron
Michael Rothery
Centre for Social Welfare Studies
Wilfrid Laurier University

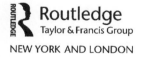
Routledge
Taylor & Francis Group

NEW YORK AND LONDON

First Published by
Lawrence Erlbaum Associates, Inc., Publishers
365 Broadway
Hillsdale, New Jersey 07642

Transferred to Digital Printing 2009 by Routledge
270 Madison Ave, New York NY 10016
27 Church Road, Hove, East Sussex, BN3 2FA

Library of Congress Cataloging-in-Publication Data

Intervening with assaulted women: current theory, research, and practice / editors,
Barbara Pressman, Gary Cameron, Michael Rothery.
      p.   cm.
      Updated papers based on presentations at a conference at Wilfrid Laurier
University in 1987.
      Includes index.
      ISBN 0-8058-0456-0
      1. Family violence—Congresses. 2. Abused women—Congresses.
3. Crisis intervention (Psychology)—Congresses. I. Pressman, Barbara M.
(Barbara Marcia), 1938–   . II. Cameron, Gary. III. Rothery, M. A., 1945–
      [DNLM: 1. Crisis intervention—congresses. 2. Violence—congresses.
3. Women—psychology—congresses. WM401 I61]
RC569.5.F3I57 1989
616.85'82—dc19
DNLM/DLC
for Library of Congress   88-38868
                                                                          CIP

Publisher's Note
The publisher has gone to great lengths to ensure the quality of this reprint
but points out that some imperfections in the original may be apparent.

Contents

Preface   vii

1
*Introduction: Implications of Assaults Against Women
for Professional Helpers*
Barbara Pressman and Michael Rothery   1

2
*Power and Ideological Issues in Intervening
With Assaulted Women*
Barbara Pressman   9

3
Treatment of Wife Abuse: The Case for Feminist Therapy
Barbara Pressman   21

4
*Family Therapy: An Approach to the Treatment
of Wife Assault*
Judith Magill   47

v

5
Effective Interventions With Assaultive Husbands
Sally E. Palmer and Ralph A. Brown   **57**

6
Effects of Family Violence on Children: New Directions
for Research and Intervention
Timothy E. Moore, Debra Pepler, Reet Mae,
and Michele Kates   **75**

7
Helping With the Termination of an Assaultive Relationship
P. Lynn McDonald   **93**
8
Transition Houses and the Problem of Family Violence
P. Lynn McDonald   **111**

9
Integrating Systems: Police, Courts, and Assaulted Women
Luke J. Fusco   **125**

10
What We Know About Preventing Wife Assault
Anne Westhues   **137**

11
Community Development Principles and Helping
Battered Women: A Summary Chapter
Gary Cameron   **157**

References   **167**
Author Index   **187**
Subject Index   **193**

Preface

*A*buse in the family is the clinical "discovery" of the past decade. Since the late 1970s, there has been a proliferation of excellent articles and books addressing wife abuse, child abuse, child sexual abuse, elder abuse, and incest survivors. This volume provides a review of the interventions to date deemed most helpful to abused women, their partners and their families as well as the theoretical underpinnings of those interventions. However, it is imperative that anyone reading this work understand that clinical intervention is not the solution to violence in the family. Therapy will only relieve the suffering of a very limited, fortunate few. Moreover, unless clinicians are knowledgeable about the causes of abuse, the impact of abuse on victims, and the issues and needs of clients traumatized by violence, victims will be thwarted in their attempts to heal themselves and victimizers will continue to endanger the emotional and physical well-being of their families.

Once compelled to respond to the problem, many therapists have attempted to treat abuse according to their familiar, respective therapeutic orientations that generally do not encompass or attend to the complexities of violence in the home. Unless the pervasive, epidemic nature of violence is recognized, a therapist may fail to appreciate that violence in the family is not a psychological problem although it maims family relationships; erodes self-esteem in women; and destroys a sense of inner strength, well-being, and trust in children. Nor is violence symptomatic of dysfunctional communication patterns, family structures, and interactional patterns. Violence in the family is a reflection of societal norms that endorse the use of violence to teach, discipline, and control; norms that exhort men to be powerful while expecting women to be pleasing and compliant; norms that diminish women and women's attributes while extolling men's attributes and power for men.

We criticize women for not leaving battering relationships, but the economic disadvantages of women render them unable to find housing or provide for their children in ways possible by remaining in abusive relationships. We expect women to leave, but membership in minority races and religions renders women unwilling to bring shame on their communities already disadvantaged by prejudice and discrimination. We expect women to nurture and protect children and hold mothers accountable when children are sexually and physically abused by their fathers, but we fail to empower women to execute the tasks we define for them and fail consistently to provide them life experiences that will enable protective, compassionate child rearing.

Unless we comprehend the social, economic, and political dimensions, and the legitimized power differentials intrinsic to violence against women and children, we will be ineffective in treating wife abuse and abuse of children. The real therapy, ultimately, is not in our offices. Ending violence against women and children necessitates significant change of the social structures that generate abusing behavior in men and designate the weakest members of the society to be the recipients of violence: women and children.

As research increasingly reveals the need for structural changes in society at large, we must be prepared for increasing "change-back" responses and backlash literature that neutralizes the painful, critical observations of our society and disparages change. This backlash has taken the form of gender-neutral descriptions of wife abuse to suggest it is a problem for which both husbands and wives are mutually responsible. It has taken the form of articles suggesting that child sexual abuse allegations are false accusations designed to prejudice courts against fathers seeking custody and, thereby, deflecting attention from the monstrously high number of substantiated child sexual abuse allegations and adult survivor reports. It has taken the form of formally organized men's groups that deny the extent of wife abuse and child sexual abuse. It has taken the form of media reports that describe the men's specious arguments, such as the low number of convicted sexual abuse perpetrators, and that fail to explain the psychological necessity for children, unsupported by parents, to retract allegations and refuse to testify against their fathers.

Unless we challenge the social structures, there are not enough therapists in the world to treat the abusers and victims who will seek our help. It is for this reason, I recommend front-line therapists become involved in activist work. By so doing, they will be addressing the source of violence in the family and will mitigate the sense of helplessness and ongoing grief and rage when continuously treating family violence. Activism can involve educating our colleagues to the complexity of wife abuse and the limitations of conventional treatment models. It can involve encouraging school boards to offer mandatory courses for both male and female students in ways to establish respectful, mutually supportive relationships; courses to develop nonviolent conflict-resolution, communication, and problem-solving skills; child-rearing courses; and courses promoting awareness that use of violence or coercion in any form is wrong. With the criminal justice system, it can involve advocacy that fosters understanding of the dynamics of wife abuse and impact on child witnesses. It can involve lobbying against pornography that not only objectifies women and children but also conveys that they relish aggressive, abusive, coercive, and painful sexuality. Only by emerging from our offices and speaking out collectively in public forums for a humane society that does not justify and legitimize inequality of women, minorities, and the poor—only then will we be working toward eradicating violence against our clients.

Barbara Pressman

Acknowledgments

This volume and its companion *Child Maltreatment : Expanding Our Concept of Helping* (Rothery & Cameron, in press) emerged from a conference on family vioence and neglect that took place in 1987 at Wilfrid Laurier University. Therefore, our acknowledgments begin by recognizing the substantial support given to this conference by the University, as well as by the Faculty of Social Work and its Dean, Dr. Shankar Yelaja. Acknowledgments are due to the conference organizing committee headed by Marilyn Jacobs. We also appreciate the valuable feedback received from the 450 colleagues from the helping professions who attended the conference. It is these people who suggested publishing not just the proceedings of the conference but rather a series of updated chapters based on the original discussions. Of course the authors also in this volume deserve our gratitude for their painstaking re-writing to often impossible editorial deadlines.

Financial support from the Ontario Ministry of Community and Social Services, the Social Sciences and Humanities Research Council, and from the Wilfrid Laurier University Research Office has made this publication possible and we are thankful for this assistance. We also recognize our considerable debt to Christine Daly and Roza Cunningham who unfailingly transcribed what we wrote and what we meant, to John McCallom who prepared the index—and to Sue Crowne for managing the logistics of the entire venture, keeping it as close to schedule as was humanly possible.

Barbara Pressman
Gary Cameron
Michael Rothery

1

Introduction: Implications of Assaults Against Women for Professional Helpers

Barbara Pressman
Michael Rothery
Wilfrid Laurier University

*O*nly recently has it been acknowledged that physical coercion, threats, and assaults against women are a significant feature of family life in our society. In retrospect, it is astonishing that those of us working in the human services—social workers, psychologists, police officers, medical workers, and the like—did not realize how many of our clients were victims of abuse. Now, with accumulating documentation indicating how distressingly common the problem is, the issue of assaults against women has far-reaching effects on how we perform our work. This book explores these impacts from several viewpoints. This introduction gives the reader a preview of the chapters, highlighting the major implications they contain for workers directly involved with abused clients.

How is it that those of us who have dealt with the consequences of wife assault and other kinds of violence against women have been blind to the extent and seriousness of this problem? A partial answer to this question is that we are part of a culture that defines domestic violence as less significant than public violence, a culture much too accepting of physical coercion or threat as a means of exercising power, and a culture that tends to explain violence in ways that blame its victims for their own misfortune. Affected by such values, we have been agonizingly slow to recognize what many of our clients have suffered: systematic intimidation, coercion, and control through actual or threatened physical and psychological attack.

If we are less blind to the issue of assaults against women today than we were in the past, it is because feminists persisted in bringing the phenomenon forward and have provided the analytical tools necessary for understanding women's experiences. At the same time, researchers have documented how pervasive the problem is. As a result, the extent to which our work inevitably involves political assumptions has been made unusually clear and the practical consequences of such an understanding have been developed in considerable detail.

The specifics of different programs and different levels of intervention may vary but they are connected by common themes that are at once practical, technical, political, and ideological in their implications. Such themes are focused on by Barbara Pressman in chapters 2 and 3.

One essential idea that Pressman draws from analyses of the problem of violence against women is that such events cannot be dismissed as unusual deviant acts. In large measure, violence against women and children has persisted in our society precisely because it does not contradict cultural norms in any fundamental way. To some degree, we have all been acculturated to perceive violence as an acceptable means of exercising control—of persuading people to do what we want them to do or punishing them for having done things we do not want them to do. Moreover, we have a history of identifying particular groups of people toward whom violent behavior is permissible as a means of exercising control: women, children, racial minorities, the poor, the mentally ill.

Another theme present in Pressman's chapters is that oppression and deprivation are different manifestations of the same underlying social arrangement: The groups against whom violence is acceptable are groups who are socially and economically disadvantaged in other ways—witness the economic inequalities that affect women and their continuing exclusion from positions of power in very many sectors of our society. This systematic disempowering is obviously closely linked to continued victimization.

As a corollary to the aforementioned we can see that violence against women (as with any oppressed group) simultaneously expresses and reinforces their disempowered state. Another corollary is that the basic problem is not simply to end violence as a behavior (although that is obviously important) but, more importantly, to alter the social arrangements that violence expresses and reinforces. Women cannot be safe when at the same time they are defined as inferior and subordinate to men.

Another important theme related to Pressman's analysis is the role that professional helpers play in perpetuating women's victimization through adherence to disempowering theories and techniques. Power is an issue that is decided at social and cultural levels, as well as at personal levels, with the personal level being, normally, of the most interest to psychotherapists. It is a goal of most psychotherapies to increase personal power by helping clients assume more control over their lives in various ways.

For women clients, however, empowerment as a goal is undermined in significant ways. When psychotherapists have aimed for improved social adjustment, they have risked promoting adaptation by women clients to the same social/familial conditions that have been oppressing them. The theories guiding work with women clients have tended to validate demeaning sexist stereotypes and to prescribe for them a highly restricted social and economic role.

Ellenberger (1970, p. 292) described three conflicting views about women that prevailed during dynamic psychology's formative years: (a) women are equal to men, (b) they are complementary to men, and (c) they are inferior to men. He further suggested that Adler argued for equality and Jung for complementarity, whereas Freud accepted the inferiority of women as a basic assumption. Of these three giants, Freud has clearly been the most influential, hence the tremendous impact on psychotherapists of ideas that attempt to rationalize women's relative power-lessness, such as female masochism, penis envy, and the idea that passivity and dependency are inherent female traits.

Psychotherapists require models that help them distinguish successful from unsuccessful adapatation, and it is unlikely that such judgments can be entirely independent of the cultural norms and values in which therapists and their theories are rooted. There is an inherent flaw in this: Inevitably, judgments about what is or is not healthy for clients are contaminated by cultural assumptions about normalcy and deviance. When the cultural assumptions in question are oppressive rather than benign, standards of psychological or interpersonal adjustment may then be unwittingly used in oppressive rather than helpful ways. With respect to women, the equation of mental health with conventional sex-role prescriptions that disadvantage women is a prime example of this. Traditionally, cultural pressures on women to exclude themselves from high-paying careers, for example, were given considerable extra weight by the psychotherapeutic establishment. A desire for economic and social independence on the part of a woman was seen to signal defects in her personality (phallic striving), and implied grave impediments to her children's proper development.

Pressman points out other damaging psychotherapeutic ideas that have in-fluenced how assaulted women have been treated: (a) male violence is strictly an expression of psychopathology, and can be treated adequately from the medical model; (b) victims play such an active role in their own victimization that it is therapeutically misguided to hold the perpetrator accountable for his behavior; and (c) that domestic violence is inherent in the family system (or the person) and can be treated strictly as a personal/familial problem without connecting it to socially prescribed power imbalances.

Finally, there is a developing countertraditional view regarding therapeutic services to assaulted women. Based on an analysis that incorporates such themes, Pressman makes the case for a feminist-sensitive approach to therapy because such an approach recognizes the cultural underpinnings of wife abuse and because it recognizes that empowerment of women in such situations must be a major treatment issue. Feminist-sensitive therapy pays particular attention to power differentials and embraces strategies that are egalitarian, nonjudgmental, noncriti-cal, and respectful of women's understanding of their own experiences. It is distinguished from many traditional approaches in its willingness to assume clear value positions and in its critique of traditional family structures. Another important difference is its recognition of victimization as an imposed reality rather than as something self-created for which the client is largely responsible.

Like established individual treatments, family systems theory and therapy have been criticized by feminist therapists. Although family systems theory provides tools for an analysis of how power and roles are allocated within families, it has eschewed any clear value position that permits identification of abuses of power. Traditionally, ideas about family health have emphasized such things as differentiation, hierarchy, and the effectiveness of the family in meeting needs, but these ideas have not emphasized equality, noncoercion, and personal account-ability. Lacking these values, the family systems framework distracted us from central issues at best. At worst it encouraged victim blaming and a perpetuation of the risk of further victimization.

In her chapter "Family therapy: An Approach to the Treatment of Wife Assault" (chapter 4), Judith Magill gives full recognition to these criticisms while arguing that the family systems approach, with certain important modifications, can still make a significant contribution to helping women in assaultive relation-ships.

Significant points of difference remain between the feminist position proposed by Pressman and Magill's family systems perspective. For example, family systems thinkers maintain that violence is a consequence of specific familial relationship patterns. In contrast, Pressman stresses that the patterns that characterize wife-abuse couples are a result of violence rather than its cause and that abusers enter relationships predisposed to abuse. Magill indicates the direction for treating wife abuse that family therapists will probably follow: Increasingly, violence will be treated as a separate and primary issue, for which the male must take responsibility. Efforts to treat the couple's relationship are only undertaken after violence has been contained.

Another important adjustment to traditional family systems theory is a modification of the basic idea of circular causality. A pure circular view of the problem implies conclusions about causality that have become increasingly unac-ceptable: An assaulted woman is as much responsible for her own victimization as the man who assaults her. The violence is seen as one move in a transactional sequence that they both create and that both are responsible for modifying. This view is giving way to one more congruent with the feminist position, in which violence is seen as a consequence of the man's personal history—a learned response to conflict—that becomes a part of the couple's patterned responses to one another.

This general position is reinforced and extended by Palmer and Brown in chapter 5, which discusses interventions with assaultive husbands. Their concise and excellent review of the major models for explaining assaultive behavior by men toward their partners concludes with a rationale for the theory they have adopted for their own research—social learning theory. The empirical evidence is clear that men who have witnessed violent behavior in their own parents' marriages are more likely to reproduce this pattern when they themselves marry. Growing up in such a context, these men have learned to think that violence and love are somehow linked, and that violence is a morally correct method for asserting control.

Such lessons in living can be easily integrated with other lessons that we all learn through socialization, especially those that prize male dominance in most areas of life.

If violence toward one's spouse is a behavior that is learned through socialization, it can be unlearned and Palmer and Brown argue that it is logical for therapists to look for ways to accomplish this with assaultive husbands. By far the most popular intervention for attempting this goal is group treatment.

Drawing extensively on the clinical and empirical literature as well as on their own research, Palmer and Brown provide a survey of fundamental issues regarding group treatment of assaultive men. These issues have clinical implications as well as implications for research, and one of the bonuses of this chapter is the care that is taken throughout to address both domains.

Social learning theory implies that marital violence is a behavioral chain linking the generations. A husband is violent in part because he was taught to be so in his own family; he is also teaching his own children to carry on the same painful tradition when they grow up and marry. Thus the study and treatment of the negative effects of marital violence on children is a crucial issue, with far-reaching implications for theory about how men become assaultive as well as for treatment that may interrupt that process in a preventive way.

Moore, Pepler, Mae, and Kates (chapter 6) draw on an impressive collective experience with clinical practice and research to enrich our understanding of the basic social learning process by which violence begets violence. It is not, they argue, simply a matter of modeling whereby a child witnesses a set of behaviors and proceeds to replicate them. A child's exposure to violence does not inevitably point him along a similar path because there are powerful mediating factors that can shape a variety of outcomes.

Moore and his colleagues describe emerging evidence that children in violent homes are affected in complex ways. Emotionally, they tend to be aggressive and distressed. Cognitively, they tend to have poor problem-solving skills especially in the realm of social problems such as conflict. They also are so attuned to anger in others that they will interpret behavior toward them as anger even when it is not. Finally, they may have a general lack of confidence in their ability to manage situations.

Thus, witnessing violence against one's mother seems to have multiple impacts, and these effects would, in combination, make sons more prone to violence themselves as adults. They will be quick to perceive conflict and slow to see nonviolent alternatives for dealing with it. However, not all violent families and not all children are the same, and the replication of violence from one generation to the next does not occur inexorably. As Moore and his co-authors point out, one of the more interesting questions presently facing researchers concerned with wife assault is how some sons manage not to follow the example of their violent fathers. Tantalizing preliminary findings are presented about factors in families and in the children themselves that mediate the transmission of violence between generations. Such information will eventually have tremendous practical importance. If, as was suggested earlier, violence is a behavioral chain, it is a chain with some weak links; the more we know about these, the better able we will be to break it. Our eventual goal in facing the problem of violence is obviously prevention and the provision of effective services to children who have witnessed violence in their parents is doubly important. Such services can meet the immediate needs of the children at the same time as they contribute to our society's long-term need to reduce the frequency of assaults against women.

In their efforts to prevent recurrence of assault at a personal level, women are faced with difficult, fundamental choices. Often their needs for self-protection require that they leave their assaultive partners at least temporarily. In chapters 7 and 8, Lynn McDonald explores the difficulties surrounding the choice to maintain or discontinue a relationship characterized by violence.

Theories about why women stay in or leave relationships in which they are physically assaulted cover a range very similar to theories about the causes of the violence itself. Some emphasize personal factors and motives, some focus on interpersonal or relationship variables, and some stress broader social and cultural factors. As with other aspects of assaults against women, a root issue is power: Whether women are able to act in their own (and their children's) best interests depends on whether they are sufficiently strong in terms of personal and social resources.

An important point raised by McDonald is that the kinds of support or empowerment required to adequately assist women who decide to terminate an abusive relationship are not a short-term proposition. Violence has such power to organize people that we become preoccupied with violent acts themselves, sometimes to the exclusion of other issues. As important as stopping violence is, helpers should not forget that the service needs of victims do not stop with the cessation of physical attacks upon them.

Whether the move out of an assaultive relationship is temporary or permanent, one support required by women to make such a decision is obvious: they and their children need somewhere safe to go. The first transition house or shelter established in recognition of this need was, as McDonald reports in chapter 8, founded in 1971. Since then, the shelter movement has undergone tremendous growth and diversification. McDonald describes the history of the movement, stressing its early ideological commitment to feminism and radical social change. As the movement has grown, different models have emerged. McDonald identifies four basic types of shelter presently operating.

Earlier, we described a tension that exists between traditional models and the feminist-sensitive perspective that has impelled some therapists to adapt feminist explanations of wife assault to their work. Interestingly, there is a parallel tension in the development of women's shelters. McDonald describes pressures on shelters (from funding bodies and other sources) to comply with traditional approaches to the delivery of social services, and it appears that sometimes the price of financial security is increased distance from the ideological traditions in which shelters are rooted.

Readers will also find much to interest them in McDonald's summary of research on shelters and their services. The demand is clear, the kinds of services they are called on to provide implies a broad and flexible role for shelters in the communities that they serve, and indications are that they have been successful in preventing recurrence of abuse for many women.

Another organizational and societal response to wife abuse has been from the criminal justice system. The police and courts are a very visible example of traditional services that have had to change in response to growing awareness of the problem of assaults against women. Because the legal system is our society's voice for declaring certain behaviors unacceptable, it can be argued that it has passively encouraged wife assault in the past. By agreeing to treat wife assault as a private familial problem, the legal system has effectively sanctioned it. In his chapter on the role of the police and courts in dealing with assaulted women, Fusco (chapter 9) documents some of the effects of this on women in the past: Women have been left unassisted and unprotected by police and court officials who have been guilty of a covert toleration of wife beating. Although women often report that calling the police is one of the most effective steps they have taken in making their partners stop being violent, they have, until recently, often been met with ambivalence.

In many jurisdictions, Fusco documents dramatic changes. Police departments have developed protocols that reinforce the responsibility of officers to investigate all complaints and to lay charges where appropriate. The result has been sharp increases in charges laid and in reports from women that this is an effective way of protecting them from future violence. Obviously, the police and courts alone cannot provide a complete solution to the problem, and Fusco discusses different models for integrating police efforts with those of other helpers. The evidence supporting the need to employ clear legal authority while remaining sensitive to the nonlegal needs of the woman and her family is unusually clear.

In her chapter on prevention, Anne Westhues (chapter 10) recapitulates issues raised in earlier chapters with respect to the impacts of different causal explanations for wife assault. Where earlier chapters show how beliefs about the roots of the problem have far-reaching effects on how service providers respond to it, Westhues focuses on prevention and the various forms it takes as a result of contending explanations for wife abuse.

The importance of looking at wife assault in ways that integrate an under-standing of the personal/familial experience with an understanding of the cultural, social, and political realities that shape that experience is a theme that is present throughout this volume. To date, the implications of such an integrated view for prevention have not been widely discussed, and Westhues' chapter therefore addresses an important gap in the literature. Particularly important, as she points out, is the hitherto understudied question of primary prevention.

Professional helpers facing the problem of assaults against women have much to learn in the process. Although the lessons to be learned are valid for work with many types of client, assaulted women present these issues with unusual clarity and force: Traditional modes of helping are insufficient in themselves and may even make helpers unwitting accessories in their clients' victimization; we cannot effectively respond to assaulted women without somehow confronting the social and political realities that support violence; we cannot help clients who are trapped in violent situations unless our goals include empowerment; our efforts to facilitate empowerment will be insufficient if we treat domestic violence as a purely private affair and restrict ourselves to a personal/familial level of analysis and intervention.

These understandings are present throughout the chapters in this book, and they are influencing how we intervene in violent situations. None of the authors, however, seem to think that the task of exploring the implications for treatment and prevention is in any sense complete. It is therefore consistent with the spirit of the volume that Gary Cameron (chapter 11) concludes with a chapter pointing to significant contradictions and areas of unfinished business. From the perspective of a community developer, professional helpers who consider that assaults against women are expressions of economic and social inferiorization and who prize empowerment as a goal perpetuate a dilemma to the extent that they continue to favor familiar professional definitions of the helping situation.

Equality implies reciprocity and this is difficult to achieve when one person is defined as an expert in relation to another. Empowerment is seldom exclusively personal; it also implies collective action and changes in the collective identity of the inferiorized group. Efforts to redress power inequalities make little sense unless they also attempt to equalize access to social and material resources. These observations, Cameron indicates, carry with them implications that have not been fully realized in the chapters of this book.

From a community change perspective, a comprehensive response to violence against women requires more than therapy. An attention to the informal helping that can occur between the women in a community is crucial. Attention must also be given to preserving the political and ideological insights that forced us to become aware of the issue in the first place but that we are in danger of losing as services to assaulted women become absorbed by mainstream professional social services. Also vital is an expansion of ideas of helping to include attention to a range of environmental supports and stressors that may be essential for a woman struggling to repair or escape from a violent relationship. Thus the book closes, appropriately, with a challenge: Can professional helpers expand their conception of their role and responsibility in ways that reflect their growing awareness that violence against women, once regarded as a private misery is also a communal problem and a communal responsibility?

2

Power and Ideological Issues in Intervening With Assaulted Women

Barbara Pressman
Wilfrid Laurier University

No therapeutic problem is more interwoven with power issues than wife abuse. No problem in a microcosm form more embodies the inequity, prejudice, and discrimination rampant in our society at large. Wife abuse reflects power differentials in our society played out in the family. It also reflects the privilege of power and authority to maintain control by means deemed acceptable by that society and the acceptable means is violence.

Friedrich and Boriskin (1982) specified that among any of the conditions that exist for child abuse to occur there is always present a cultural tolerance for severe corporal punishment. This view is reiterated by Steele and Pollock (1974). In their extensive study of abusive parents, they concluded that "in dealing with the abused child we are not observing an isolated, unique phenomenon, but only the extensive form of what we would call a pattern or style of child rearing quite prevalent in our culture" (p. 90).

Dobash and Dobash (1977-1978) pointed out that all legal systems in Europe, England, and early America supported a husband's right to beat his wife. Community norms did so as well. In 18th-century France, for example, it was considered fitting for a husband to chastise his wife for reasons such as assertion of her independence, wanting to retain control of her property after marriage, adultery, or even suspected infidelity. However, the beatings were supposed to conform to the rules of legitimate punishment. The chastisement of wives, like that of children, was restricted to "blows, thumps, kicks or punches on the back . . . which did not leave any marks" (Dobash & Dobash, 1977–1978, p. 430).

Laws permitting and/or describing acceptable physical ways to punish wives existed for many centuries before the repeal of such laws barely 100 years ago. The attempts to modify the belief that wife beating is an unacceptable norm are barely 10 years old.

DISCRIMINATION AGAINST WOMEN
IN THE PRESENT

When I describe wife abuse as reflecting the severe inequality of women in our society, there may be some who question this statement and argue that women have entered formerly male-dominated occupations. Women have acquired the right to vote and to own property. They can even smoke in public. Despite all these acquired rights, there exists much prejudice against women and denial of equal opportunity. A few of the institutionalized practices that maintain women as second-class citizens are described in the following pages.

Labor

The work of women is downgraded by prevalent societal myths regarding the role of women in the labor force. These myths are the basis for discriminatory practices against women and unequal treatment in the marketplace. It is believed, for example, that the contribution made by working women to the economy and to their families is less important than that of working men. The implication here is that women workers are not genuinely dependent on their incomes and, therefore, do not unduly suffer if unemployed. They are labeled secondary workers. The facts, however, eradicate the myth: Thirty-nine percent of all working women in Ontario are single, widowed, or divorced. These women are working to support themselves and, in many cases, dependents as well (Statistics Canada, 1985). Women working outside of the home who are members of two-parent families make a contribution equally essential. Were these women to leave the labor force, it is estimated that the number of poor families in Canada would almost double (National Council of Welfare, 1979).

Although full-time employed women earn 62% of what men earn (Statistics Canada, 1977), this does not mean that their wages are not essential. The salaries, not the women, are secondary. Even for occupations where the majority of workers are female, women receive lower pay than their male counterparts.

Education

Although girls perform as successfully and frequently with higher grades than boys at the elementary school level, female motivation and aspiration drop sharply in high school. The Report of the Royal Commission on the Status of Women (1970) cites childrearing practices and family values as highly relevant in effective educational motivation for children. If training a child to be independent and self-reliant is an encouragement to high achievement, the reverse will be true as well. The Commission also cites the paucity of inspirational models for women as a deterrent to high achievement. Men in high positions in business and public life serve as models for boys, but there are few models for girls.

Further examples of the discrimination against women to achieve are illustrated by financial arrangements for university men and women. A survey by the Dominion Bureau of Statistics (cited in Report of the Royal Commission, 1970) indicates that there is no substantial difference between the essential expenses of men and women students. However, despite the same percentages of men and women receiving scholarships and grants, men receive proportionately higher aggregate sums of money than those obtained by women.

Media

Numerous studies cited in James Doyle's (1983) *The Male Experience* all conclude that television depicts men either as heroes or villains and women as either adulators or victims. Television commercials also convey stereotyped images of gender roles. In general, women are portrayed as domestics who are concerned primarily with household problems. Doyle (1983) said, "The underlying message is that women are concerned only with their physical attributes, preservation of their beauty, and delay of the aging process, and men are interested only in power, status and achievement" (p. 98).

SOURCES OF DISCRIMINATION

In my classes, I have found students from minority groups identifying with women's experiences. They recognize that women experience treatment comparable to that of minorities and immigrants. Indeed, women are afforded minority status in our society.

I emphasize and highlight cultural and attitudinal causes sustaining wife abuse because how we define the causes will determine how we approach and treat the problem. There are those who would argue that there is a high incidence of alcoholism present in wife abuse, and frequently there is. However, alcoholism is not the cause. Anne Ganley (1981), who worked extensively with abusing men, found that 25% never drink; 25% are social drinkers (never become intoxicated); 25% abuse only when drunk; and 25% abuse when drunk or sober.

Moreover, wife abuse is not caused by skill deficits such as the inability to communicate adequately or to control the explosive expression of anger, because abusing men do not usually direct their anger at others. Their anger and pejorative, denigrating words are directed exclusively at their partners.   Their physical violence, too, is confined to partners. The ability to confine the expression of anger and physical violence suggests a great capacity to control themselves.   Furthermore, some men consciously do not use their fists but carefully use the flat of their hands and consciously choose where on the body they strike their wives. The anger and violence become means by which these men control their partners, and their right to maintain that control is an integral part of our social structure.   Gondolf and Russell (1986) found that it is relatively easy to end the use of physical violence by anger management programs; however, the use of other controlling mechanisms such as verbal abuse, restrictions on the use of the family car, and unilateral decision making concerning finances persist.   Gondolf and Russell also found that when abuse and control of women in its many forms ended, men had changed in three areas: willingness to share decision making, development of a changed definition of maleness, development of an empathic understanding of a mate's experiences.

INTERVENTION

The Political Dimension of Therapy

In light of these findings and in light of the extensive literature describing women's experiences that result in feelings of both powerlessness and lack of control over their own lives, treatment of wife abuse must involve men learning to share power and decision making and women becoming empowered. To redress the inequities experienced by all women, not just abused women, empowerment of women and raising their awareness of the relationship of their feelings of depression, anxiety and low self-esteem with their second-class status are critical.

When lecturing on women's problems, the link of those problems with oppression, and the need to empower women through therapy, I have been asked whether or not I am being political. My response is that I am being political, and I make no apologies for my political stance, which is openly declared and explained. I believe that all therapy is potentially political; however, most therapists do not recognize this potential. By political, I am referring not merely to the science of government but also to the science of power and the structure of power in our society. The existing structure affords privilege and status to men and disfranchisement for women. Examples of this disfranchisement, historically and in the present, were cited earlier. I would add to the meaning of political, the measures that respect and maintain the existing power structure and the measures that oppose it.

The Politics of Beliefs About Women

How we view wife abuse is not only relevant for addressing power differentials between husband and wives in therapy, but it also raises an issue of power in the realm of therapeutic models and ideas. I am referring to ideas that have become so entrenched in our way of viewing clients that these ideas have taken on a power of their own. Sociologist Dorothy Smith (1975) described two elements of the power of ideas: (a) those that gain wide appeal because they conform to and confirm prevailing social structures, and (b) those that become so widely accepted that they resist change in light of refuting research findings. In other words, ideas become autonomous agents in society, independent of those who think them and of the actual practical situations in which the particular thought arises and to which it is relevant. Freudian concepts have taken on such a power in our society. The characterization—or I should say character assassination—of women as masochistic, passive, morally inferior to men and envious of the male genital organ has been disproved by the research of Caplan (1987), Masson (1985), Masters and Johnson (1966), and many others. However, Freudian views regarding women resist modification. Consequently, those embracing a traditional therapeutic orientation misinterpret women's behavior, diagnose erroneously and treat symptoms not the impact of underlying life experiences. Examples of this misapplication are particularly likely to occur with the following groups: women who extricate themselves from one battering relationship and marry subsequent batterers, and incest survivors who marry abusive partners. It is an easy and logical deduction to conclude that these situations are evidence of female masochism and women's need for continual pain. The conclusion, however, is inaccurate, for it fails to acknowledge the impact of abusive experiences on these women and the consequent gravitation to very needy men. Abusing men generally suffer very low self-esteem and a history of abuse in childhood (Rosenbaum & O'Leary, 1981a); Roy, 1982), which deprived them of the nurturing and emotional support they subsequently seek in partners. Abused women, and women in general, are socialized to believe they are responsible for caregiving and emotionally supporting all family members. Incest survivors were parentified children; that is, children who performed adult roles in the family. They were expected not only to perform and help with household chores but also to take responsibility for those tasks. Other forms of parentification include serving as a sexual partner for the father and protecting the mother by maintaining secrecy (Gelinas, 1983). As a parentified child, the incest survivor becomes especially sensitive to the belief that it is her role to be a caregiver. Consequently, she will tend to choose a man for whom caretaking is particularly important (Gelinas, 1983). It is not masochistic pain that abused women seek. Repeated abuse is often indicative of a very caregiving, nurturing woman attracting a very needy man and abusing men are among the neediest of men.

Another misunderstood group of women are those who remain in battering relationships. Again, the remaining is not an indicator of female masochism but rather deeply imbedded social values and expectations of women that predispose them to stay in abusive relationships.

Any therapist who believes that a battered woman has the choice to leave the field that is hurtful to her is making a judgment based on a number of tacit assumptions about women, some of which are listed here.

- Women are willing and able to attend to their own needs for safety, freedom from verbal abuse, and for nurturing relationships even if these needs conflict with their partners' needs.

- Women can attend to their own needs despite their belief that children need their biological fathers as long as they are not abusing their children or acting unkindly to them.

- Women are able to see themselves functioning independently of others, especially partners.

- If women do not have the economic potential to maintain for their children the quality of life afforded by remaining with their partners, women can view the economic losses as secondary in the face of their need for safety.

- If women are economically disadvantaged by leaving an abusive relationship, they have the competitive qualities and career aspirations necessary to restore economic stability for their children.

To determine whether these assumptions hold any validity, one must examine the writings of those who extensively counsel women and those both studying women's experiences and summarizing recent research into women's lives. The consistent findings of these authors offers compelling evidence to refute the previously stated assumptions that have no foundation in women's actual experience or socialization.

Jean Baker Miller (1986) found that women are not encouraged to develop their unique potential. "Instead, they are encouraged to concentrate on forming and maintaining a relationship to one person" (p. 18). Furthermore, women are taught that if they were to pursue intellectual and skill-building endeavors, there would be disastrous consequences: "They will forfeit the possibility of having any close relationships" (p. 19). Consequently, women come to view their needs "as if they were identical to those of others—usually men or children" (p. 19).

Reviewing the socialization studies of males and females, Penfold and Walker (1983) concluded that girls are programmed to think that their primary achievement is to be wives and mothers.

Rewarded for social achievement not objective achievement as they mature, girls and women know their worth only from others' responses and their identities only from their relationships as daughters, girlfriends, wives, or mothers (Bardwick

2. Power and Ideological Issues

& Douvan, 1972). Bardwick and Douvan cited research with female college students in regard to what would make them happy or unhappy and when they would consider themselves successful. Both undergraduate and graduate students gave the same reply. "When I love and am loved; when I contribute to the welfare of others; when I have established a good family life and have happy, normal children; when I know I have created a good, rewarding stable relationship" (Bardwick & Douvan, 1972, p. 231).

Reviewing the research of Matina Horner, Carol Gilligan (1982) described women as experiencing anxiety about competitive achievement. Women's difficulty with competitive achievement "seemed to emanate from a perceived conflict between femininity and success" (Gilligan, 1982, p. 14). For women, the anticipated negative consequences of success, especially achievement involving competition with men, are the threat of social rejection and loss of femininity.

The Politics of the Therapeutic Relationship

When therapists are uninformed and ignorant of current research regarding wife abuse, and when they treat abused women who remain in battering relationships or are ambivalent about leaving as masochistic, they are being political. When therapists are uninformed and ignorant of current research regarding female psychology and when they ignore the social, economic, and political context in which women live, they are also being political. In communicating to women a therapeutic judgment stating that their continued involvement in battering relationships is masochistic, therapists become political for they impose on their clients myths about women that depict women as intrinsically psychologically flawed and, therefore, inferior. Adopting the masochistic view of women indicates therapists who have no appreciation or recognition of the impact of social norms and the impact of victimization trauma on the functioning of women. Subscribing to theories that view women as inferior and masochistic becomes political because those views justify the existing social structure. This political act may not be conscious. These values regarding women are so ingrained, they are not even thought about or questioned. As therapists, we must become conscious of the ways in which our understanding of human behavior reflects cultural values rather than actual human experiences.

Women's studies programs and women's courses are a major step toward recognizing that there is a history peculiar to women: a history of oppression and a history of persistent, painful revolution by increments rather than by upheaval; revolution by constant civil agitation, lobbying and education rather than disobedience and violence. There is a history of women's achievements in spite of discrimination, ridicule, and denigration. There is also a recognition in women's courses, especially women's psychology courses, of the dreadful cost to women's emotional well-being because of that discrimination and denigration. However, unless such ideas and information permeate mainstream psychology and therapy programs, there will exist the ongoing danger that women presenting problems and symptoms will be misunderstood, misdiagnosed, and mistreated. All too often, women's issues and dissatisfactions are regarded by the mainstream therapeutic community as faddish or as a reflection of female pathology. Thereby, therapy unwittingly becomes a tool to maintain the status quo rather than challenge the destructive prevailing order.

When therapists in general talk of domestic violence or spousal abuse and the issue before them is wife assault, this description becomes a political act whereby the violence of the husband is neutralized, and the wife becomes responsible for the abuse against her. Violence in the family is not gender neutral nor is it randomly distributed. Violence in the family is perpetrated against those who are weak and those who are perceived as weak: Violence in the family is directed at women, children, and the elderly.

The work of Shirley Endicott Small (1981) documents the fact that most marital violence is directed against women by men. She stated that 60% of all female homicide victims are killed in a family context; a figure that is more than double the percentage of male victims killed in similar situations. Moreover, Statistics Canada (1982) states that although two-fifths of all homicides in Canada are between spouses, the vast majority of the victims are women. Those women who do kill their husbands are usually acting in self-defense.

Another model that is unwittingly political is family systems therapy. Family systems therapy has been especially criticized by feminist therapists (Avis, 1988; Bograd, 1984; Pressman, 1989) for its neutral orientation and failure to appreciate the social, economic, and political elements of society that affect women. Furthermore, systems therapy adheres to a model that dismisses causes of behavior as irrelevant and focuses on interactional patterns by family members that perpetuate and mutually reinforce dysfunctional behavior in the family. It is a theory of problem maintenance, not of causality (Watzlawick, Weakland, & Fisch, 1974). Thereby, women are indirectly blamed for their own victimization, and male perpetrators of violence are not held accountable for their violence.

Reviewing the literature that examines attitudes toward women in therapy, Avis (1988) found subtle biases in family systems theory that result in attributing responsibility to women for family problems as well as responsibility for affecting change. This tendency exists despite the pride family therapy takes in itself for employing a blameless notion of systemic interaction where there are no victims and no villains. She further pointed out the subtle biased assumptions underlying much of family therapy practices; for example, that it is primarily women's responsibility for childrearing. Consequently, children's problems are attributed principally to inadequacies in mothers. Although there is emphasis on engaging fathers in family therapy, involvement of fathers is aimed at helping mothers out or teaching mothers more effective parenting skills.

A parallel finding was documented by Caplan and Hall-McCorquodale (1985). In their study of nine major clinical journals over a 3-year period, they found mother-blaming prevalent in all nine journals and most strongly so in *Family*

Process, a prominent family therapy journal. Caplan and Hall-McCorquodale documented a tendency in clinical journals to idealize fathers, to describe them in only positive terms, and not to see their behavior or lack of specific behaviors as contributing to their children's difficulties.

Finally, a repeated theme in family therapy practice is the unchallenged reinforcement of stereotyped sex roles (Avis, 1988; Bograd, 1984). The acceptance of traditional relationship arrangements as the ideal fails to appreciate the consequences of traditional socialization for women. This socialization renders women feeling helpless, dependent, and passive. Thereby, its promotion becomes a political act, for therapists again unwittingly endorse expectations of women that will reinforce their sense of inadequacy and powerlessness.

Thus far, I have described two issues of power related to wife abuse. First, this phenomenon is a reflection of inequitable social norms and redressing these norms necessitates empowering women. Second, therapists hold the power to determine the cause and meaning of this symptomatic behavior and by such determinations they may: (a) wrongly hold wives responsible for their own abuse, (b) wrongly blame women for their own abuse, (c) label women in pejorative ways, or (d) fail to recognize the root causes of violence. In all of these situations, women's reality is distorted and the social norms are maintained.

A third power issue is a value-taking role. This role necessitates therapists saying that not only is violence wrong, but also it will not be tolerated. Probation officers and child protection workers take such a role. I believe, furthermore, that it is appropriate and necessary for therapists in general to take on such a role. Part of disseminating values is mandating therapy and the use of legal authority to ensure human rights and protection (i.e., safety in the home).

Therapy and Legal Sanctions Against Violence

Recently, the law has become quite clear on this matter and has enforced its power by making culpable and responsible any perpetrator of a violent act. Men who abuse their partners engage in much blaming and ruminating about their partners' misdeeds. However, it is irrelevant, before the law, that a wife did not make supper on time or did not pick up groceries that day or had not cleaned the kitchen floor or stored away the children's toys. If therapists are caught up in the wife's behavior, which indeed may not be angelic, and give substance to the belief that she plays a role in her husband's violence, abusing men will continue to blame their wives. They will not recognize that the issue is the nature of their responses to events they do not like or want.

Invoking the power of legal authority may seem to be an anathema to many therapists trained to respect the right of clients to determine their own life courses. However, this view is questionable when the individual's behavior constitutes a threat to others or when his or her own life is at risk. A husband announcing his intention to hurt his wife, a child at risk of abuse, and clients talking of suicide are all instances in which therapists have the responsibility to fulfill advocacy and protection roles. They have the responsibility to maintain protective roles for those who cannot protect themselves. It is a difficult balancing act to treat the one who has committed the endangering acts while maintaining cognizance of those who are at risk. I believe that this awareness must be maintained in order that we may help both perpetrators and violent clients to take responsibility for their acts and help them to develop an empathic understanding of the pain and harm they inflict. With abusing men, that empathic response is essential in ending the use of further violence (Gondolf & Russell, 1986). The balancing act for the therapist is maintaining a sense of the humanity of the abuser while recognizing the pain of the victim.

It has become clear from the research of Giarretto (1976) and Finkelhor (1984) that the power of the law is a critical element in the treatment of perpetrators of child sexual abuse. That power has also proven to be highly relevant in diminishing wife abuse (Burris & Jaffe, 1983). Violence and controlling behavior has its rewards: compliant wives and the release of tensions. Arrest, trial, public exposure, and actual or potential imprisonment are all powerful deterrents and negative sanctions to counteract the immediate gratification of acting–out power and maintaining control of others via violence.

Dispowerment and Secrecy: The Therapist's Response

Another dimension of self-determination is that of allowing clients to decide when to raise topics for therapy. Therapists frequently suggest that clients will initiate certain material when they are ready to do so. Therapists initiating charged material are viewed as disrespectful and intrusive. This view, I believe, fails to differentiate between the clients' right to pursue a specific area and the responsibility of the therapist to convey that he or she is one with whom the client can discuss any event or subject. By raising very difficult subjects—history of incest, child sexual abuse, sexual assault in adulthood, and wife abuse—the therapist conveys that he or she will not be overwhelmed or revolted by the recounting of such experiences. By raising such topics, he or she can convey to clients that they will not be criticized for any life experiences, for their families' responses to these events or for their coping strategies.

Violence is the best kept secret in our society. Clients will maintain this secrecy just as carefully in therapeutic situations as in other life interactions. Although battered women seek help from doctors and counselors for a variety of concerns, violence is not a concern they reveal although it may be the one that underlies all the others. Among incest survivors as well, victims tend to seek psychiatric treatment without disclosing their early sexual abuse. Instead, they usually show characteristic symptomatic behaviors. These behaviors duplicate the symptoms of the borderline personality. If these symptoms are the focus of treatment, therapy tends to be relatively unsuccessful. When these symptoms are treated as the direct result of incestuous experiences, therapy is highly successful (Gelinas, 1983). The reader should be cautioned that talking of one form of violence with clients will not elicit talk of another. Therefore, each form of violence must specifically be a focus of inquiry.

By not raising emotionally charged subjects, a therapist (a) colludes in the client's maintaining secrecy, (b) implies to the client that some subjects are so painful they cannot be tolerated either by the client or therapist, and (c) conveys that some subjects are so distasteful and offensive that to discuss them would only repel the therapist and contaminate the relationship between therapist and client. Finally, by maintaining secrecy, we as therapists further isolate clients already isolated by their pain and suffering. Not only do we isolate them but also we deprive them of any possibility of validating how hurtful their early experiences were and of providing comfort. By maintaining silence, we deprive clients of the opportunity to examine the source of their suffering and symptoms and to establish new understanding of that symptomatic behavior. This new understanding needs to be based not on self-blame, self-contempt, and distorted perceptions of their symptoms, but on the relationship between classic coping strategies and responses and the traumatic experience of abuse.

CONCLUSION

In this chapter, I have attempted to illustrate how therapy is a political arena. I suggested further that neutrality in therapy is a myth. I urge, therefore, that we become conscious of our values in order that what we convey in therapy does not empower one group of people at the expense of another. Finally, I wish to make it clear that in becoming sensitive to the way therapy has tended to discredit, blame, and denigrate women while exalting men, I am not advocating hostility toward men. All too often a feminist perspective becomes equated with hostile, antagonistic, bitter, bra-burning women. I think—I certainly hope—that the many men I have counseled and continue to counsel have experienced fairness and genuine concern with me. Just as I oppose social injunctions that favor men at the expense of women, I oppose behaviors that denigrate men to promote women. What I am advocating is equality for men and women both in therapy and in society at large. What I am advocating are therapeutic practices that empower human beings and give them control over his or her own respective lives. I am advocating practices that very carefully integrate knowledge of the social context of the human experience into our understanding of human behavior.

3

Treatment of Wife Abuse: The Case for Feminist Therapy

Barbara Pressman
Wilfrid Laurier University

*T*o treat wife abuse effectively, I believe it is critical to understand the root causes of wife abuse and the corresponding issues for husbands and wives; issues that must be addressed in order to restore the well-being of each family member and to insure the safety of all family members. Wife abuse is such a pervasive and frequent occurrence that explanations exploring only couple and family interactional patterns or describing individual partners in terms of pathological symptomatology ignore the fact that statistically violence against wives is almost a norm. Wife abuse occurs in every socioeconomic, religious, and cultural group (Dobash & Dobash, 1979; McCormick, 1981). Furthermore, according to Canadian estimates based on known statistics—police records, doctors' reports, social work records, clergymen's accounts—one woman in eight is physically abused by her partner (MacLeod, 1987). A thorough and comprehensive study in the United States by Straus, Gelles, and Steinmetz (1980) cites that figure as being one woman in six. If one includes psychological and emotional assaults such as intimidation and verbal denigration, that figure would expand significantly. In fact, many shelters include verbal and emotional abuse alone as prerequisites for admittance.

Wife abuse is a reflection of societal norms and attitudes. Its elimination necessitates the cooperative efforts of all our social institutions; that is, the medical community, government, labor, religious organizations, schools, and the criminal justice system, as well as social services. The focus of this chapter is on the therapeutic community. The purpose is to (a) detail behavioral patterns of each family member, the structure present in wife-abused families and consequent treatment issues; (b) examine the shortcomings of the theoretical orientations and respective treatment approaches of a number of therapeutic models when applied to wife abuse; (c) propose a theoretical framework that encompasses the complexity of wife abuse; and (d) describe a treatment format evolving from the theoretical model proposed.

FAMILY STRUCTURE AND PATTERNS OF BEHAVIOR IN WIFE-ABUSED FAMILIES

The Abuser

When a husband physically abuses his wife, he is also always verbally abusive. Numerous times, battered women have said "I'd rather he hit me a dozen times than once hear the things he says. The bruises heal, but I can never forget the words."

Wives are often accused of being sluts, of being unappealing, of being incompetent housekeepers and inadequate mothers. The attacks focus on those areas of their lives that are most relevant to a sense of self-worth and those aspects of life whereby they measure themselves as successful women: homemaking, child care, attractiveness, sexual appeal and fidelity. These are the norms of a successful woman in our society, norms that they accept and to which they aspire.

Not only does the husband verbally denigrate his wife, but he also undermines her role with their children both by criticizing her in front of them and by actively telling the children they do not need to obey her directives (Pressman, 1987).

Of the men who abuse their partners, 80% come from homes in which they were abused, or in which they observed their mothers being abused (Rosenbaum & O'Leary, 1981a; Roy, 1982). Consequently, the batterer's early life experiences typically are characterized by the lack of a nurturing father. His father was viewed as frightening and nonprotective, and his mother was experienced as unable to protect him or herself. Deprived of a loving, protective environment, the batterer did not learn to trust others. He became an adult unable to trust other adults, including his wife. Early emotional deprivation renders him also as one who is very needy of nurturance and support. Consequently, the batterer expects enormous, unrealistic sustenance from his partner to make him feel good about himself. Because the battering husband lacks self-esteem, fears losing his partner, and is jealous of her relationships with other people, including relatives, he tends actively to discourage his partner's relationships with other people. He accomplishes his isolation of her by acting inhospitable to her guests, demeaning them, criticizing them to her, and displaying intense rancour, displeasure and anger at his wife's desire for contact. To avoid the tension and strife in their homes, battered wives defer to their husbands' wishes to end or severely limit other relationships. Not only is the abuser an isolated human being, ultimately, the abuser also isolates his partner and becomes the primary, if not sole source of adult companionship and support for her.

Characteristic too of the abuser are very stereotyped, traditional views of gender roles (Gondolf, 1985c). To him, real men are the breadwinners and ultimate decision makers with little responsibility for the emotional climate of the family. Consistent with these stereotypes is the belief that real men are strong, dominant, superior, and successful (Trimble, 1986). Feelings of inadequacy in any of these areas were found to be devastating to the batterer's self-esteem (Coleman, 1980).

In short, battering men use control in many forms (withholding money, regulating the use of the family vehicle, verbal intimidation, denigration, and violence) as a means of getting their needs met. Maintaining the image of men as strong, unemotional, self-reliant as well as lacking trust; the batterer tends to have superficial contacts and friendships with others. When he does have close friends, he tends not to share with them his problems or discuss deep, personal feelings (Ganley, 1981).

The Battered Woman

Denied relationships outside the home and ashamed to talk of her abuse when she does have contacts, a battered woman lacks support for her situation and realistic feedback regarding the horror of her abuse experiences. As a consequence of the isolation imposed by her partner, the battered woman may turn to her children for emotional support and comfort, thereby, she propels her children into an adult role. Even when able to fulfill a disciplining role in the family, a battered woman frequently is overly protective and shies away from being punitive or demanding of her children. Recognizing that her children are pained by the father's explosive outbursts, she attempts to maintain a special closeness with them and to protect them from disciplinary acts that she perceives as sources of further pain and hardship. In this way, she believes she is balancing the harshness of the father.

To deal with the horror of the abuse, a battered woman may involuntarily experience psychic numbing; that is, she becomes emotionally withdrawn and affectively deadened. This numbing and depression, which is common to abused women, may render her unable to be available to her children for guidance, for emotional support, and even for their physical well-being (Pressman, 1984).

Each battered woman feels ashamed of the abuse against her because, like most women whether abused or not, she functions by the societal rule that holds women responsible for the emotional well-being of all family members. Therefore, should family members be unhappy or act inappropriately, she believes she must be to blame.

Not only does the battered woman blame herself and not only does her partner blame her, but the helping professions also blames her, and women in general, for family problems (Pressman, 1984). The tendency to blame mothers for the problems of their children is well documented by Caplan and Hall-McCorquodale (1985). Holding the woman in the home responsible for the dysfunctional behavior of children is the therapeutic bias by which professionals powerfully reinforce the expectation that women be responsible for the behavior of others in the home (Avis, 1988).

When a woman does recognize that her husband has a problem and that she is not the cause of the violence, she still maintains silence about her situation to protect him from being criticized or ostracized by the community or family members. She also believes that as a caregiver she should help her troubled partner. Frequently, battered women who disclose to therapists, do so in order to learn how to become better wives who do not provoke such behavior in their partners or to learn how to help their husbands with their problems.

In short, battered women believe that if they were satisfactory wives, if they could only get it right, then their husbands would not abuse them. Consequently, compliance is a major characteristic of battered women and a major survival technique to meet their partners' needs, to maintain the belief that they have control over his behavior and the means of avoiding further abuse. Because the battered woman is not successful in ending the abuse, because she is isolated and lacks adequate support, generally, she is depressed.

Children From Wife-Abused Homes

Even when the mother does not actively turn to her children as an emotional resource, in their sensitivity to her suffering, children very often comfort and soothe her.   In horror, during a meeting of a woman's support group, I watched a 2-year-old crawl into her crying mother's lap, reach out a tiny hand to stroke her mother's cheek and croon, "No cry, mommy; make it better. It be all right." Instead of thanking the child and indicating that she would be all right and that she had the support of group members to comfort her and that the child could continue playing, the mother responded by clinging to the child and accepting her solace. In that moment, the child lost her childhood and all the essential dependency, protection, and security childhood should embody. She became an adult fulfilling the nurturing role to an agonized child–mother.

In general, child witnesses of abuse evidence the same symptoms as children who are directly abused (Jaffe, Wolfe, Wilson, & Zak, 1986b). They believe they are to blame for the abuse of the mother, believe they should be able to help their parents, feel powerless, suffer low self-esteem, frequently become aggressive (boys) or withdrawn (girls), are depressed, often achieve poorly in school and are truant, suffer isolation, and learn that violence is an acceptable norm (Elbow, 1982; Moore, Pepler, Mae, & Kates, chapter 6, this volume; Sopp-Gilson, 1980). Male children frequently repeat the pattern of abuse in adulthood, and female children learn that compliance and meeting other's needs are the ways to survive and achieve acceptance (Rosenbaum & O'Leary, 1981a). To summarize, the impact of witnessing abuse constitutes severe emotional damage and trauma for children. It damages ability to trust, decimates self-esteem, and distorts values. Violence becomes acceptable and normal behavior in relationships, a problem-solving tool, and an insured way for men to have their needs met.

Family Structure

The following is a description of the family structure and the emotional cycle present once violence against a wife occurs. In no way is it an explanation for the violence because this structure emanates from and does not necessarily precede violence (Pressman, 1989).

- The husband is controlling in order to get his needs met.

- The wife is demoted in the executive, adult hierarchy and, because of the abuse, emotionally withdraws from him. She may do all his bidding and try to please him; however, because of the verbal and physical assaults and fear, she cannot feel close.

- The husband isolates his partner from friends, relatives, and contacts outside the family.

- The children are parentified, indulged, or neglected and become equals to mother. They try to protect and/or comfort her.

- The husband feels more isolated, lonely, and becomes more controlling.

- In general, the family is isolated from community involvement and outside resources. Children are reluctant to bring friends home (Pressman, 1984).

- A major family rule is maintaining secrecy about the violence. It is quite common for battered women to seek help from clergymen, doctors, and counselors; however, they do not identify violence as the central problem or even as a factor in their lives (Pressman, 1987). Common presenting problems of abused women or wife-abused couples are the wife's depression, communication, the wife's anxiety, and dissatisfaction with the sexual component of the marriage.

- The husband believes that he cannot live without his partner and is often suicidal when his wife leaves or talks of leaving. The wife believes she cannot leave him because he will hurt himself or be unable to survive without her. In time, she may lose any sense of her strength or confidence in her ability to care for herself such that she believes she cannot survive without him. Consequently, there is a symbiotic quality to the wife-abused couple.

- The structure described here (father aggressive and controlling, mother dependent and compliant) is one of the two major types of families A. Nicholas Groth (1982) described as characteristic of incest families. Frequently, shelter workers detect symptoms of child sexual abuse in the children housed in their shelters (Pressman, 1987).

TREATMENT ISSUES

The preceding section provides a description of the husbands' predisposition to abusive behavior before entering marriage and a description of women's and children's responses to and ways of coping with the abuse. As well, the interactional patterns and the role of socialization and traditional gender roles have been outlined. Based on this understanding of individual family members and their functioning as a family, family members will be confronting the following issues.

Battered Women

- Attending to their own safety; recognizing they are responsible for and have a right to care for themselves; and developing safety resources and strategies.
- Recognizing they are not to blame for the violence of others.
- Ending denial and minimization of the violence as a coping strategy to endure the pain and horror of abuse.
- When deciding to remain with abusive partners, developing coping strategies that are not self-destructive or hurtful to children (drinking, drug abuse, withdrawal, turning to children) but that afford support, safety, and enhanced self-esteem (talking with friends, taking skill or job-training courses, attending a women's support group, ending the secrecy).
- Dispelling and challenging the societal myths and expectations of women, which blame women for remaining in battering relationships while supporting that they do so.
- Developing an awareness of their strengths, skills, and competence.
- Re-establishing the sense of power over their own lives and overcoming the belief that they are helpless and powerless.
- Developing the sense of self-worth by recognizing they have the right both to express their own needs and to satisfy them.

- Making a connection between low self-esteem, depression, and societal rules that delegate women to second-class status and that demand that they put all others before themselves.

- Recognizing feelings of helplessness and connecting those feelings with the experience of being abused; with the socialization of women; with the social and economic context that discriminates against and oppresses women; with a possible history of physical or sexual abuse as a child.

- Establishing a social network whereby the isolation and family secrecy are overcome.

- Developing a broader view of male–female roles, interactions, and characteristics.

- Learning to express feelings regarding victimization especially rage and anger without feeling inhuman, unfeminine, and disloyal.

- Recognizing and articulating the ambivalence regarding abusers who are not monsters, are not always abusive, and who possess many endearing qualities.

- Dealing with grief and loss should they separate.

- Recognizing they have the capacity to be family executives whether in the relationship or not; recognizing however, that unless their husbands get help, they will never function as equals or respected adults in the home.

Child Witnesses of Wife Abuse

- Learning norms of behavior regarding violence: Violence is wrong.

- Dealing with ambivalence about the abuser.

- Mourning when mother separates from father.

- Dealing with the denigrating words of father regarding mother, especially when parents are separated and children visit father.

- Helping mother be open with the children regarding her decision to leave and her reasons for leaving.

- Role modeling of male–female relationships that are not gender stereotyped by male–female group co-leaders.

- Learning appropriate expression of feelings rather than withdrawal or aggression.

- Individuating when children are fused with mother; learning appropriate child role as opposed to parentified child who is support to parents.

- Gaining self-esteem.

- Learning to trust.

- Dealing with feelings of guilt that he or she is responsible for causing the violence and/or for preventing it.

- Establishing safety resources.

- Addressing abandonment fears.

- Addressing feelings of helplessness.

- Exploring possible sexual abuse.

- Dealing with depression and the possibility of suicide.

- Expanding support networks for stability (school personnel, Big Brothers, YM/WCA, etc.).

Abusing Men

- Ending the denial and minimization of violence out of shame and as a means to avoid facing the pain they inflict on partners.

- Taking responsibility for violent behavior and being accountable for that violence by openly acknowledging it; by no longer trying to justify it; by actively trying to end the use of violence against partners without expecting rewards, wife's approval of their return as acknowledgement of change; by adhering to wife's wishes to end contact; by recognizing that violence is only one of many means by which men attempt to control partners.

- Making connections between early experiences of abuse and current behavior as a means of developing an empathic response to abused women and as a way of recognizing that abuse was a pattern they learned prior to knowing his wife who is not, therefore, responsible for the abusive behavior.

- Developing motivation to seek help other than fear of imprisonment or loss of partners.

- Developing a view of male–female roles whereby women are equal, not subordinate to men, and whereby men can express a range of feelings without seeing themselves as feminine but human.

- Developing trust in others.

- Establishing a support network whereby they can continue to explore the values and attitudes examined in group; whereby they can end the enormous dependence on partners for emotional support, and whereby they will receive support from and expectation from other men to be non-violent.

- Developing a sense of self-worth that is not predicated on controlling anyone else but having control over their own being; that is not predicated on having to fight to be men; that is not predicated on being a winner and evidencing achievement or productivity but on being human beings with intrinsic value and innate dignity.

- Recognizing that battering men frequently are depressed and prone to suicide when partners leave or threaten to leave.

- No longer experiencing jealousy and a need to isolate a partner from other relationships.

- Sharing decision making with partners, not hearing differences of opinion as challenges to their authority or signs of disrespect.

FAILURE OF THREE MODELS TO ADDRESS WIFE ABUSE: TRADITIONAL–PSYCHODYNAMIC, FAMILY SYSTEMS THERAPY, PSYCHOEDUCATIONAL GROUPS

Any model treating wife abuse must address the issues described here. The following models (a) fail to address many of the identified issues; (b) exacerbate many of the issues; (c) subtly blame the victim; and/or (d) do not insist that abusers become accountable for abusive behavior.

Traditional–Psychodynamic Therapy

Illustrative of the weaknesses in traditional therapy is the following case study:

A woman requested an appointment with me at the recommendation of her lawyer. Although she had been in therapy for several months with another therapist, the lawyer urged her to see me because of my work with abused women. She had been married for 13 years, had two children (aged 10 and 12), and had been separated for 2 years. When I asked what the focus of therapy had been, she stated that she and the therapist were constantly dealing with crises precipitated by her husband who continually contravened recommendations about custody and visitation as a means of maintaining control and thwarting the wife's wishes and requests. Her position was reactive, and

she felt she had no control over her own life. She was depressed, lacked any
sense of power, tried not to cry in front of her children lest she appear weak,
firmly believed that her responsibility was uniquely to her children and that
their needs held priority in her life.

To determine what she would like to achieve from therapy, I asked what
goals she wished to establish. She stated she would like her children to know
that violence is wrong and is not to be tolerated, and her daughter to know she
need not remain in a battering relationship as she had done for 13 years. Upon
hearing these goals, I asked the woman what she did for herself. She looked
startled, puzzled, and disoriented by my question, and stated that she did
nothing for herself. She went on to say, "How can I do for myself, when I
don't even know what I want for myself?" I suggested that by exclusively
serving others, her children could not appreciate that not only does she have
needs, but also that her needs count. Her son would learn to expect women
to serve him; and her daughter, to expect that her role is primarily to serve
others. When I asked her to consider the possibility of meeting her needs some
of the time, she responded that such behavior would be selfish.

This woman exemplified total acceptance of the caregiving role prescribed for
women to the detriment of herself and the view that showing emotion equates with
weakness. Because the consulting client experienced her therapist as caring and
respectful and wished to continue with her, I suggested that the focus of their work
might be recognizing that she has a right and responsibility to care for herself in
addition to others. The means for caring for herself would be identifying what her
needs and goals are and how to achieve these. The thrust of therapy I was proposing
was no longer reactive, but goal oriented and indicated my belief in her ability to
take charge of her own life. My proposal aimed at empowering this woman and
broadening her view of caregiving to include herself.

Focus on Pathology Within the Individual

Although supportive, this woman's therapist did not take into account the
ingrained values and life experiences of women that render them likely to remain
in battering relationships; likely to gravitate to future battering partners and servile
relationships; or that cause them to feel inadequate, inferior, powerless and,
therefore, depressed. Traditional therapy dismisses and distorts the reality of
oppressive experiences for women; thwarts the empowerment of women; and
labels common presenting symptoms in women as pathologic rather than the only
conceivable response to demeaning, overwhelming, and traumatic life events
(Chesler, 1973; Greenspan, 1983; Nairne & Smith, 1985).

Frequently, abused women, like nonabused women, seek the help of
psychiatrists, counselors, or medical doctors for depression, anxiety, fatigue,
complaints regarding abdominal pain, gastro-intestinal disorders, backaches,
headaches, and sleep disorders. Using the medical model, symptomatic behavior
that does not have organic roots is regarded as emotional illness. When women
who embrace accepted, traditional roles suffer discontent they are labeled as

pathological for not experiencing satisfaction in the ways expected of them and deemed fulfilling (Chesler, 1973; Nairne & Smith, 1985). In this scheme, there is no recognition of the imposition of a second-class status on women nor of the impact of economic dependence and the fear engendered by believing that one cannot cope on one's own. There is no recognition of the impact of controlling partners who do not permit wives to have access to family cars or to share in decisions regarding family finances. There is no recognition of the impact of being solely responsible for household chores and children while often being expected to work outside of the home as well.

There is also no regard for a woman's experience of being abused, for all too often doctors and psychiatrists do not inquire about women's ongoing experiences and marital relationships. Many of my abused clients and those of other therapists (Meade-Ramrattan, Cerre, & Porto, 1980) have been treated for depression with drugs or shock treatment. No one asked about their marriages; nor about level of satisfaction regarding communication, sexual experience, affection, decision making and noncouple friendships. No one asked how they resolved differences and expressed anger with each other. No one asked when anger was expressed, did anyone get slapped or pushed or kicked or had hair pulled or were things thrown about or walls punched or kicked. If there had been such questions and answers indicating dissatisfaction and/or violence, the woman's symptoms of depression (often anger one fears expressing and, therefore, turns inward), anxiety, sleep disturbances, and eating disorders (signs of masked depression) might be viewed as logical responses to feeling no power in one's life, fear, and isolation. Until therapists ask questions that reveal the context of a woman's life, adaptive behavioral responses to that context will continue to be interpreted as pathologic sympotomatology.

Failure to Incorporate Current Findings
Regarding Human Behavior

Not only does traditional therapy ignore women's reality but also it distorts that reality. Freud based his theory of human personality on the Oedipus complex, castration fears, penis envy and his belief that boys and girls between 3 and 5 are cognizant of the absence or presence of a penis in girls and boys respectively. He held that women are naturally (biologically and anatomically) passive, dependent, and inferior (Freud, 1959, 1965). His disciple, Deutsch (1944), painstakingly described how female reproductive anatomy inevitably makes women passive, masochistic, and weak and she corroborated Freud's previous thinking.

The research of Conn and Kanner (1947) cogently demonstrated that male children 4 to 6 years old do not even know that girls do not have penises, and that those who did know were not traumatized by this awareness. The research of Katcher (1955) confirmed this data. Although this and other recent research has challenged and discredited many of Freud's theories concerning women (Weisstein, 1972), his views in the face of this evidence continue to prevail and form the basis on which assessments and treatment plans for women are being made.

When describing abusing men, traditional therapy is also found wanting, for researchers have found that they cannot be characterized as mentally ill (Langley & Levy, 1977). In fact, battering men come from every stratum of society and are involved in every occupation (Davidson, 1978; Martin, 1976). They appear normal in all areas of functioning other than their marital relationships. They even tend to be steadily employed or may even own their own businesses (Geller, 1978).

Insight—The Basis for Change

Despite the successful functioning of batterers in many areas of their lives, traditional therapists have diagnosed them within a variety of specific dysfunctional personality types. Adams (1988), who works extensively with abusing men, is highly critical of therapy that focuses on these personality traits and intrapsychic phenomena rather than directly on the violence. Although there is much value in attending to intrapsychic factors, such as fear of abandonment, dependency, low self-esteem, or impaired ego functioning, the social sanctions for the control of women are ignored by traditional therapy. Moreover, Adams pointed out, whatever the contribution of unmet childhood needs to violence and whatever the intrapsychic factors, focusing on these does not help abusers end their violent behaviors. The violence does not end because it continues to be the means through which abusers gain compliance. Furthermore, the violence itself increases the men's feelings of insecurity and low self-esteem because abusive behavior increases the risk of wives' leaving and emotionally distances them from their husbands.

Not only is categorizing abusing men along specific personality traits ineffective for ending abuse but also the aim of traditional therapy, insight, is ineffective (Adams, 1988; Star, 1983). Men who make the connections between early life experiences and current behavior do not necessarily change. In fact, ruminating about observed parental behavior potentially affords abusers the opportunity to blame others for their violence. At the outset of therapy, it is their tendency to blame others, their wives in particular, for their abusive acts (Pressman, 1987). Therefore, a critical component in counseling abusing men rests in helping them take responsibility for their own behavior and guarding against their transferring blame to other sources such as parents or the women's movement.

Family Systems Theory

Under the directorship of Salvador Minuchin, the Philadelphia Child Guidance Center has been a major training unit for Structural Family Therapy. To illustrate structural family therapy concepts, the Center has videotaped Minuchin consulting with families. In the tape "Taming Monsters" (described in Minuchin & Fishman,

1981) parents of two daughters, ages 2 and 4, have sought help from the Center because they cannot control the behavior of their 4-year-old. After working with another therapist for five sessions, Minuchin in the tape was brought in to consult. To help the mother and father experience the pliable child dimension of the 4-year-old instead of an overwhelming out-of-control, difficult child, Minuchin established a parent–child play enactment. From the enactment, Minuchin observed the father to be gentle, involved, and sensitive to his child. However, two questions persist for him. (a) What makes being firm so difficult for mother? Even speaking firmly, loudly, or forcefully feels excessive to her. She welcomes the father's assistance and yet is critical of his harsh tone and sees him as inadequately sensitive to their children's feelings and experiences. (b) Why does each parent keep the other incompetent?

Minuchin dismissed the child from the session and worked solely with the parents. After an enactment in which the mother conveyed that the father is not sensitive enough to their children's needs and feelings and the father indicated that the mother is too soft, Minuchin was still perplexed by the aforementioned questions.

Minuchin: Asks the husband why his wife thinks he is such a tough person and he indicates his wife's need to be flexible is her response to experiencing him as so rigid. Minuchin then tells the father that he does not see him as rigid but as quite flexible and again he asks why his wife sees him as rigid and lacking understanding of children.
Husband: States that frequently he loses his temper.
Minuchin: Queries, "So what? So does she." He then reminds father of his flexible, nonauthoritarian style when playing with their daughter moments before. Minuchin asks again why his wife sees him as rigid and authoritarian.
Husband: Repeats that he loses his temper with the daughters.
Wife: Adds that he does have a short fuse.
Minuchin: Dismisses the concern and states the wife's image of him is strange. He invites another enactment in which the husband is to discuss with his wife how it is that she needs to protect the children from his short fuse. Minuchin begins the dialogue with the statement "I think she's wrong."

In this series of exchanges, both parents have alluded to a sign of violence (father's temper). However, Minuchin ignored this reference by not exploring a concern of both, minimized the concern by stating that mother has a short temper too, and totally dismissed the reality of both by telling the wife that her perception of husband is wrong.

Wife: States outright that she fears her husband's losing his temper at the girls because she has observed outbursts of temper. She expresses her fear for the children if ever he were to hit them. Also, out of her concern

about his temper, she is leaning over backwards to show them that not
everyone has a short fuse.

Father: Points out that the children will see her as backing them against him and
that they will be forming a special unit.

Minuchin: Becomes very excited at father's insight and asks him to repeat it.

As noted previously in this chapter, it is common for mothers, abused by
partners or fearful of violence and the pain the children experience, to align with
the children. In this exchange, Minuchin blamed mother rather than recognizing
her behavior as the response of fear and an attempt to provide legitimate protection.
He failed to confront father about the fear he is generating in his wife and children.
Instead, he applauded father's awareness while ignoring mother's.

Minuchin: Again asks the husband why the wife is afraid of his temper. In a
mocking tone (which later Minuchin acknowledges was jokingly
stated), he queries whether or not the husband had ever smacked his wife
and when had been the last time he beat her.

Husband: States he has never beaten his wife.

Minuchin: States that the wife talks as though she were beaten regularly.

Wife: Interjects, that she has seen the temper and that she experiences her
husband as totally out of control when his temper takes over.

Minuchin: Finally responding to her fear, asks about the temper and what articles,
such as furniture, dishes, windows, have been destroyed.

Husband: Describes the worst incidence involving hitting a wall.

Wife: Interjects that he put his fist through the wall once, and has thrown a
shoe.

Minuchin: Queries at whom the shoe was thrown.

Husband: Answers that the shoe was thrown at a wall.

Minuchin: Asks whether or not the husband's fist really penetrated a wall.

Husband: Indicates that the wall was only dented.

Minuchin: Describes to the couple that the extent to which the husband discharges
anger involves no destruction of anything.

In this exchange, Minuchin again totally dismissed the experience of fear
engendered in the wife by acts of violence: throwing objects, punching a wall. Not
only has he dismissed her fears but he has also totally minimized the violence.
Although no object was overtly broken, trust and the wife's sense of safety and her
children's safety were extensively damaged. Minuchin has failed also to acknowledge the intensity of anger evidenced by someone merely denting a wall.

Husband: In response to Minuchin's statement that nothing had been broken, the
husband replies that there is a reason for his controlling himself from
breaking objects. When he was a child his father used to tear the house

apart. He had vowed never to repeat this behavior, for he had seen it happen and . . . .

Minuchin: Cuts him off and states that what the wife fears is something that does not exist.

Wife: Again she interjects and states those events are imbedded in her memory; "They're locked in your memory."

Minuchin: Corrects her and states these events are locked in *her* memory.

Wife: Agrees with him and reiterates that those memories are the reason she fears her husband. Again she states how well she is aware of the extent to which her husband can be out of control.

Minuchin: Responds by telling the husband that his wife is talking of a myth, and a bag of lies, which he urges the husband not to believe. He expands the metaphor by telling the husband the wife is selling him the idea regarding his temper, his rigidity, and his destructiveness. The most the husband may be is stronger than the wife, nothing more.

Wife: Upon hearing this evaluation of her, the wife states that Minuchin's assessment frightens her.

So forcefully has Minuchin presented his case that the wife is now questioning her own view and is alarmed by *her* distortion and unfairness to her husband.

Minuchin: Ends the session by reiterating that the wife's image of her husband is distorted and that he expected the husband to have struck her once or twice on the basis of her expressed fear. He concludes by asking the husband why his wife thinks he could hurt his daughters when, "You are soft as a teddy bear."

Not only did Minuchin disregard the wife's fears, he also dismissed the husband's reality and early experiences of abuse. By not focusing on the husband's experience of pain as a child, Minuchin missed an important opportunity to help the husband empathically respond both to his wife's fears and his children's, for they have witnessed in him what he witnessed in his father. That the father is soft is only one dimension of his personality and is not unique within violent husbands. The expectation too that her fear was justified only if she had been actively assaulted reflects a complete lack of comprehension of the experience of those who witness violent acts and hear intensely angry words. They experience fear, anxiety, uncertainty, and constant watchfulness in anticipation of, and in readiness to avoid further such episodes.

Circular Causality

This tape demonstrates several concepts of family systems theory that are destructive when applied to family violence: circular causality, neutrality, and inattention to the traumatic impact of human experience. According to family systems theory, why a problem situation exists is irrelevant to what the situation is because explanation "usually contributes nothing toward its solution" (Watzlawick, Weakland, & Fisch, 1974, p. 86). Developers of family systems theory experienced the tenacity with which families engaged in particular behaviors that sustained presenting problems. Consequently, family dysfunctioning is viewed as the consequence of problem maintenance: The wife's perception of her husband as rigid, harsh, and potentially hurtful generates her flexibility, vigilance, and protectiveness that in turn generates the father's rigidity and harshness. There is no provision in systems theory for questions concerning causality, nor a focus on early history that may contribute to current family behaviors (Minuchin 1974).

The underlying premise of many family systems therapists when working with wife abuse is that the violence is not the key issue. Instead, the family structure and interactional patterns are the significant problem (Bograd, 1984). "What triggers it [violence], however, is not evil triumphing over good, but a sequence of interpersonal events" (Minuchin, 1984, p. 177). This premise totally ignores the fact that more than 80% of abusers (Rosenbaum & O'Leary, 1981a; Roy, 1982) were abused as children or witnessed abuse and come into relationships predisposed to be abusive (Pressman, 1987). The focal issue, I believe, is the violence from which dysfunctional family interactions and structure evolve.

By focusing on circular interactional patterns, the wife is subtly blamed for sustaining the husband's violent behavior and is, therefore, deemed responsible for her own victimization (Bograd, 1984; Goldner, 1985b). Moreover, according to the systemic view of the family, the family is an open system that operates as a whole. To change one part of the family, therefore, influences change in the entire system (Watzlawick, Beavin, & Jackson, 1967). However, when a husband is violent, a compliant wife becoming defiant will still be abused and a defiant wife becoming compliant will also be abused. Only the husband's ending his violence will afford the abused wife an environment in which she can change in relation to her husband.

Neutrality

This concept implies that all family members are equally responsible for maintaining dysfunctional behavioral patterns (Watzlawick et al., 1974). Therefore, neutrality suggests that each family member, including children, is equally powerful. This position totally ignores cultural and economic realities that render women disadvantaged regarding economic autonomy, power, and status within the family (Dobash & Dobash, 1977–1978; Nairne & Smith, 1985). It further disguises the mammoth power differentials between adults and children that exist because children are dependent on parents for survival.

By holding all family members responsible for dysfunctional behavior such as violence, neutrality holds no one member accountable, including the one who employs violence. In *Family Kaleidoscope*, Minuchin (1984) even questioned how therapists can intervene if they focus on the violent act. He believed that focusing attention on the man "as monster" (p. 175) will only invite defensive aggression in response to aggression. He assumed that therapists confronting abusing men about unacceptable behavior and helping them to accept responsibility for that behavior is tantamount to vilifying them as monsters. Therapists engaging abusing men in therapy to end violence and other controlling behaviors, are able to focus on the violence while conveying sensitivity to the men's pain at this behavior and to their struggle with a most distressing human problem. In short, therapists focusing on violence are able to embrace the human being while conveying the unacceptability of violent behavior. To pursue Minuchin's neutral stance would result in ignoring child abuse and sexual abuse in the home lest a systems therapist blame the perpetrator.

Absence of Attention to Trauma and Intrapsychic Functioning

In fact, a case example cited in *Family Kaleidoscope*, is that of a child who was struck so severely by her father when she intervened to help her abused mother that hospitalization was required and permanent hearing impairment in one ear was possible. Not focusing on the violence can only result in the abused individual concluding that his or her abuse experiences are minor and insignificant. The abused can only feel abandoned and experience distortion of their reality. This case is also a glaring example of the reluctance to deal not only with the physical dangers of abuse but also with the emotional damage resulting from abuse. The emotional scarring of children who have witnessed their mothers' abuse has been carefully documented and cited earlier in this chapter.

The traumatic impact of abuse on women has also been well documented (Martin, 1976; Pressman, 1984; Star, 1980; Walker, 1977–78) and is evidenced by anxiety, fear, psychosomatic disorders, depression, lowered self-esteem, and a sense of total helplessness and powerlessness over one's own life.

Although the work of Bowen (1978) and Framo (1976) is highly respected, much of the family systems therapy literature describes interventions that focus on present interactional patterns rather than on the consequences of events that are traumatic to intrapsychic functioning. Consequently, an increasing number of therapists are expressing concern that family systems therapy does not address the internal, personal pain of individual family members. They are documenting that change solely in family interactions and structure is insufficient to help many individuals overcome the impact of traumatic family events and deal with their own internal suffering (Grunebaum & Belfer, 1986; Nichols, 1987; Schwartz, 1987).

Moreover, family systems therapists who focus exclusively on the here and now, do not help abusing men deal with their own childhood victimization that has contributed to their abusing behavior. It is essential that they examine the way this early abuse affects their current functioning and behavior.

Treating the Marital Subsystem Together to Address Wife Abuse

The literature advocating couple therapy to treat wife abuse (Cook & Frantz-Cook, 1984; Geller & Wasserstrom, 1984; Magill & Werk, 1985; Margolin, 1979; Taylor, 1984) emphasizes treatment that generally is psychoeducational in nature. The therapists help the husband and wife recognize cues to his becoming violent; track interactional patterns that precede violent behavior; and stress communication skills and anger management. Although these approaches may effectively reduce violence for the time being, they do not explore the cultural stereotypes and norms that expect and then reinforce men to take on the male postures and attitudes that underlie wife abuse (Brennan, 1985; Gondolf & Russell, 1986; Saunders, 1984).

Furthermore, therapists who initiate couple work for wife-abused couples predicated on a judgment that mild violence does not necessitate individual work first are perpetuating the mythology that there are mild as opposed to severe forms of violence. The attitudes and values that generate all forms are the same.

A request for marital counseling when violence against the wife exists and when the couple wishes to reside together does not necessitate conjoint therapy. Nor is separate counseling inconsistent with their goals for an improved marriage. Weakland (1983) insisted that one can think systemically while not seeing all members of the system together. He then highlighted the usefulnes of separate work to redress dysfunctional complementary relationships (i.e., excessively helpful family member and needy member).

Although it is the responsibility of the therapist to acknowledge the clients' stated goals, the means is also the responsibility of the therapist. If individual work to correct a power imbalance by helping the husband end the use of violence is the treatment of choice, the therapist must indicate this and state how separate work in groups will help the couple toward attaining their goal of an improved marital relationship. The therapist can stress how the violence is hurting the relationship, distances the wife, and deprives both of the connectedness they desire. It is my experience that most couples agree to this recommendation.

Group Counseling

Psychoeducational Focus

Although there are a growing number of programs for abusing men (Star, 1983), researchers (Adams, 1988; Gondolf & Russell, 1986; Jennings, 1987) are becoming increasingly concerned that programs are exclusively focusing on psychoeducational issues; namely, stress reduction techniques, identification of cues to anger before anger builds to explosive proportions; cognitive restructuring or rewriting internal scripts that intensify anger (Ganley, 1981; Purdy & Nickle,

1981); and relaxation exercises. Although these programs may successfully end physical violence, the research suggests they do not end verbal abuse (Brennan, 1985; Gondolf & Russell, 1986). Unless violence and anger are recognized as only two of the many mechanisms by which husbands control partners, control of women will persist by those who had been physically violent. Therapists with a feminist orientation toward treating abusing men view violence against women as a means of control and focus on the men maintaining journals documenting episodes of controlling behavior rather than anger logs. Another dimension of such groups is consciousness raising for men to help them make the connections between their controlling behavior and the social forces and expectations of men that endorse such control. Gondolf and Russell (1986) have found that when control of wives is not the focus of therapy, violence and control in the form of verbal debasement persists even though physical violence may abate. Those men who ended the use of controlling behaviors as well as violence changed in three significant areas: redefinition of manhood, willingness to share decision making with partners, and newly developed empathic response to a wife's experience of and feelings regarding abuse. Group programs that stress skill deficits may help end the physical violence; however, "the attitudes that maintained the violence continued much longer" (Brennan, 1985, p.651) and generated continued coercive, controlling behavior and resulted in damaged marital relationships.

Often group programs stressing skill development are structured in format. Men who are abusive gain a specious sense of power by controlling wives. They, therefore, need to develop a sense of power in their lives predicated not on controlling others but on strength and competence from within. If the leaders determine what the program content will be each week, an important opportunity for men to ask for what they need and to learn that their contributions are important is lost. Although the men will need the skills taught in a structured program, it is my experience and that of Jennings (1987) that men will themselves raise the topics that will spontaneously precipitate a focus on skill development. Moreover, the client determining what he needs to change in himself allows him to take responsibility for behaviors he views as interfering with satisfaction in his life rather than blame others. Jennings found that the unstructured format enhances the possibility for the men to address issues outlined in this chapter. An unstructured open group also encourages the men to teach one another what they have learned, affords ample opportunity for men to support and nurture one another, and allows members to hear and, therefore, appreciate different points of view and different perspectives. A prescribed, formally constructed, didactic program is not conducive to men developing self-reliance, self-directedness, ownership of their own struggles, and access to themselves for solutions and support.

Nature of Leadership for Both Men and Women

A further contentious issue among leaders of groups for abusing men and battered women is the nature of leadership. The argument has been advanced that men should be leading men's groups and women should be leading women's groups or there should be male–female co-leadership in both men's and women's groups. Male–female co-leadership for men permits a broadened view of male–female roles and behaviors. A male–female leadership team provides an opportunity for a male and female to model equality; to model intermittent deferring respectively of the one to the other; to model each asking the advice of the other at different times; and occasionally provides leadership exclusively by one or the other. The men also are able to witness a man and woman mutually supporting each other in a nurturing, affectionate and nonsexual way. Often the men in my groups believe that male–female relationships can only be sexual and that all touch is erotic.

The argument I advance for exclusively female leadership of the women's group is quite different. Those who propose male–female leadership for the women's group believe that women too need such models of men deferring to women and views of men different from the ones they have experienced. However, women's attitudes toward men are significantly different from those of men toward women. Not all women who have been abused by partners were abused as children or witnessed controlling fathers. They do not necessarily view men negatively or as inferior. On the contrary, they view men very favorably, even too favorably. A reluctance to leave abusing partners derives from their fears of being alone and of not being able to manage without a man. It is not men they view negatively but themselves and their own capacity to rely on and care for themselves. Because women view themselves in such pejorative terms, it is critical that they have models of women in positions of leadership, women who convey both confidence in themselves and a belief in women's potential.

Negative cultural attitudes toward women and discrimination against women cited in chapter 2 are ingrained not only in men who hold privileged status but also in women who have come to view their own contributions and potential as inferior to that of men. Smith (1975) cogently described the limited number of models of women in managerial positions in education and cited numerous studies documenting that college women are prejudiced against what women academics and women writers say. What men have to say is regarded as more important and more authoritative than what women have to say. To counter such prejudice and doubt regarding other women, entirely female leadership of women's groups is essential lest valued ideas generated by the female co-leader be attributed to the male co-leader. Given the social context, women, and most especially battered women, need to learn that they are capable of holding positions of responsibility, are capable of making decisions, and are capable of being the source of their own strength. This strength is innate, intrinsic, and not the gift of any other human being. It must never be viewed as deriving from a male giving them permission to be strong but from their own awareness of the worth of all women and the right of all women to express and experience their own inborn gifts and competence.

Closed Group and Finite Number of Sessions

There are compelling arguments for closed groups: (a) the increased potential for cohesion and closeness among members, and (b) the opportunity for very structured movement and growth phases. However, there are decided advantages to open groups: (a) old members provide role models for advocating nonviolent marital relationship and readily challenge new members' attempts to justify violence or controlling behaviors with wives; (b) old members who have learned nonviolent, nonintimidating communication styles become the teachers of the new members; (c) old members model openness in expressing feelings and concern for others; and (d) old members who have changed offer hope to new members that change is possible (Pressman, 1984).

With respect to the number of sessions, I suggest for both the men's and women's groups a contract of goals and a specific timeframe. Although the men's group contract is aimed to end the use of violence and control of women, the men, like the women, are encouraged to define their own goals in their respective group. Members of each group are asked to make a commitment for a specific number of sessions. The number of sessions varies for different organizations from 6 to 12. From my work with battered women, I believe that a minimum of 12 sessions is required to help most women regain a sense of their own worth and capacity to attend to their own needs. For women who had experienced abuse as children or who have experienced abuse in their marriages for many years, the time required may be much longer. Therefore, I believe the women themselves are the ones to determine the amount of time they need in the group to meet their goals. Most women I have counseled remained in the group for 6 months. A very small percentage (between 1% and 5%) required a year or more. Invariably, the women who remained longest, during sessions to assess whether or not their goals had been met, said they needed the support of the group to affirm their strength and provide support while they were extricating themselves from partners who continued to harass them. Other women needing protracted time had chosen to remain in abusive marriages. These women did not receive support from family or friends who thought they were mad to remain with their husbands. These women attended group despite bitter opposition by their partners for doing so. Attendance was the one way they nurtured themselves, declared needs in opposition to their partner's needs, and provided a nurturing environment for themselves.

Because the men in the men's group are working to change attitudes and values so deeply ingrained they are almost visceral and because there is virtually no support outside of the group for these new values and ways of thinking, I believe men require a minimum of 6 months in their group. Research (e.g., Adams, 1981; Brennan, 1985) confirms the need for lengthy counseling.

Because it is relatively easy to end the use of violence against women in a brief time and because government funding agencies may gravitate to the least expensive form of treatment, I urge therapists undertaking these programs to be mindful of the necessity for long-term counseling and for the necessity to attend not only to overt violence, but also to all those means by which husbands intimidate, control, and demean their partners.

PROPOSED THEORETICAL FRAMEWORK

The theoretical orientation of feminist-sensitive therapy is the recognition of the impact of social, political, and economic norms (some of which have been described earlier in this volume) on the emotional well-being of women (Greenspan, 1985). Feminist-sensitive therapy makes the connection between social, political, and economic discrimination against women and the corresponding injury to women in the form of low self-esteem, depression, anxiety, somatic complaints, sleeping problems, and eating disorders (Nairne & Smith, 1985). Feminist-sensitive therapy further recognizes that the epidemic number of assaults against women (rape, wife abuse, and incest) is not a function of intrinsic pathology in women or men, nor a function of circular, mutually reinforcing behavioral patterns of husband and wives (Minuchin, 1984). These are, in fact, tragic reflections of the economic, political, and cultural norms that endorse and legitimize the view of women as inferior and subordinate and which condone the use of violence against women (Brownmiller, 1975; Dobash & Dobash, 1979).

Feminist-sensitive therapy holds that the emotional well-being of women can improve primarily by their becoming aware of the relationship between these experiences and their presenting problems; and the relationship between what they have been taught to believe about themselves as women and how they feel about their own self-worth as individuals.

Effective counseling for abused women and battering husbands must take into account not only the economic, political, and social context in which they live but also the prevailing attitudes and expectations regarding gender roles. Only by understanding the social context, gender roles, and socialized traits can therapists begin to comprehend why men abuse their partners, why women remain in battering relationships, and why women feel powerless, helpless, and less competent than men to take charge of their own lives.

Although very clear principles have been delineated by feminist therapists and writers (Greenspan, 1983; Penfold & Walker, 1983; Rawlings & Carter, 1977; Wyckoff, 1977), these principles do not preclude the incorporation of other theoretical models to explain human behavior nor a range of interventions from other theoretical models to achieve client goals.

The traditional psychoanalytic view of men and women reflects the enormous influence of cultural norms rather than inherent human characteristics. The explanation that male–female traits are based on penis envy and Oedipal resolution, and much of the theoretical tenets of traditional psychoanalysis have been disproved. In spite of early inaccurate conclusions, a psychoanalytic lens to view behavior and personality development as a function of childrearing experiences and parent–child interactions can be highly useful. Chodorow (1978) has successfully formulated a psychoanalytic understanding of the development of the female persona that is ultimately a reproduction of the oppressive social order. As well, Miller (1986) integrated a psychodynamic understanding of women with an acutely sensitive feminist perspective. The work of Avis (1988) describes ways to integrate feminist therapy principles and family systems therapy. Recognizing the need for women to ventilate anger at oppressive and abusive experiences, Greenspan (1983) advocated Gestalt techniques to help women purge themselves of their rage.

Whatever other theoretical models feminist therapists employ, the feminist therapist is ever cognizant of the role of oppression and denigration in the lives of women. Consequently, feminist therapists strive to: (a) eliminate authoritarian, intimidating behavior in therapy, (b) empower women by helping them become aware that they have choices in and control over their own lives, and (c) help women become acquainted with their unique strengths and worth. In short, feminist therapy is not a series of specific techniques. It is a perspective, a way of seeing and understanding the context in which women live (Penfold & Walker, 1983; Wyckoff, 1977). To ensure that these aims are not contaminated, feminist therapists translate them into specific principles and strategies.

Principles of Feminist Therapy

1. Commitment to the view that men and women are intrinsically equal and possess equal potential to men; that women have the right to declare and fulfill their inherent potential; and that it is wrong for women to be subordinate to men.
2. Awareness of the necessity of bringing a feminist analysis to each woman's current situation.
3. Grounding in current research about women.
4. Egalitarian approach to therapy with a careful avoidance of placing the client in a one-down position from the therapist.
5. Recognition of the importance of the female therapist as a role model for women clients.
6. Willingness of the therapist to spell out his or her own values to women seeking their guidance.
7. Willingness of the therapist to make use of self-disclosure as it relates to shared experiences.
8. Centering therapeutic strategies around maintenance and enhancement of women's power.
9. General, incorporation of sex-role analysis, with a comparison of the costs and benefits of traditional and feminist values.
10. Maintaining open files to the client who may join her therapist in writing progress notes or reports which might be required by outside agencies.

11. In family work, helping families to recognize and change the destructive consequences of stereotyped roles and expectations in the family.

12. Avoiding the promotion of dependency.

13. Emphasis on client's strength and competence.

14. In family or couple work, giving equal consideration to the skills, aspirations and careers of women rather than viewing women as weak, dependent and inadequate and their career goals secondary to partners.

15. Avoidance of fostering or reinforcing guilt or blame.(This does not mean that women are not helped to appreciate their responsibility for particular behavior patterns or are not confronted on behavioral contradictions.)

16. Offering therapeutic perceptions as opinions expressed in behavioral terms rather than as pronouncements about what is really going on (Avis, 1988; Brody, 1984; Greenspan, 1983; Penfold & Walker, 1983; Rawlings & Carter, 1977; Rohrbaugh, 1979).

Strategies in Feminist Therapy to Fulfill Principles

1. The woman establishes her own goals and objectives in the form of a contract with the therapist and has a right to determine the number of sessions she wishes to attend. Moreover, the client decides how she will attain those goals.

2. Group counseling is the preferred mode of therapy, for it dilutes the client's dependency on the therapist and encourages trusting, helpful relationships with other women.

3. The language of therapy reflects the equality of the relationship: (a) client rather than patient is preferred; (b) psychological jargon and esoteric clinical explanations of behavior are avoided; and (c) therapists are addressed by first names.

4. A part of therapy may involve teaching women skills such as stress management and assertiveness.

CONCLUSIONS

The work of Dobash and Dobash (1979), Adams (1988), Gil (1986), and Gondolf and Russell (1986) conclude that wife abuse is a reflection of cultural norms and institutionalized inequities regarding male–female roles, behaviors, and opportunities. The epidemic proportions of violence against women is further evidence of the sociological conditions endemic to our society, which foster violent behavior against women. As soon as one accepts this conclusion, one has embraced the feminist perspective.

The childhood experiences of batterers and the social learning of cultural values in their families of origin predispose them to the control of partners, unrealistic expectations of partners, self-doubt, and jealousy. The potential for violence precedes the relationship and cannot be explained as a function of interactional patterns between partners (Pressman, 1987). Social learning and the internalization of cultural norms in women predisposes them to remain in battering relationships and feel responsible for the abuse perpetrated by partners. The issues present in wife abuse revolve around two major themes:

- The battering men's need to be in control of partners must be abandoned and stereotyped views of manhood must be questioned and challenged in order for abuse of women to end.

- The abused women's sense of powerlessness must be replaced by a sense of control over their own lives and the inculcated belief that women are responsible for the emotional well-being of all family members and are, therefore, to blame for any problems arising in individual members must be challenged and replaced by recognizing that violence is the responsibility of the abuser.

It is critical to address the causes outlined here; to treat the traumatic effects on men of early abuse and for those men who have not been abused; to challenge the internalized stereotyped values that permit control of wives. To explore the many issues described above, separate group work for men, women, and children is required.

Major elements of feminist therapy are: the sex-role analysis of the problem, separate counseling for abused and abusers; recognition of the necessity to redistribute power between husbands and wives, and to redefine manhood and womanhood. To treat a wife-abused couple without addressing power and control issues and without examining gender roles, not only fails to explore focal issues, but also puts wives at risk of further abuse. From my own experience and that of colleagues treating wife-abused couples who had experienced couple therapy before individual work, there is a common report from these couples. When violence was not the focus of couple therapy, violence did not end. When violence was the focus, but not control by husbands, verbal abuse and denigration persisted as did other forms of controlling behavior.

Finally, in light of the internalized experience of powerlessness, helplessness, and worthlessness of abused women, therapy for women must not further erode their sense of self-esteem and control over their own lives. The tenets and strategies of feminist therapy ensure respect for women's view of their experiences, appreciates women's competence and strength, and heightens women's awareness of their worth and that of women in general. Feminist therapy principles are, therefore, especially relevant, appropriate and essential to address the many issues of wife abuse and serve the needs of battered women.

4

Family Therapy: An Approach to the Treatment of Wife Assault

Judith Magill
McGill University

*T*he role of family therapy in dealing with wife abuse is a subject of current debate and polarized views. Although wife battering has not been addressed in major works of the family systems literature (Bograd, 1984), systemic writers and clinicians are beginning to develop theories and clinical interventions to respond to male violence against women in the family. These responses have ranged from traditional ones viewing the violence as a symptom of the dysfunctional system and not addressing it directly (Minuchin, 1984); to attempts to develop new formulations and models of intervention that give special status and meaning to the violence (Bagarozzi & Giddings, 1983; Cook & Frantz-Cook, 1984; Giles-Sims, 1983; Taylor, 1984). These latter formulations represent important developments in family therapy as it faces issues like wife abuse, child abuse, and incest.

Feminist thinkers (Bograd, 1984; MacKinnon & Miller, 1987) have criticized systemic approaches to wife battering as constituting another form of victim blaming, perpetuating the unequal distribution of power based on gender, and for not acknowledging the differential processes of socialization that maintain the imbalance of power. Most models of family therapy are seen by feminists as conservative, reinforcing the status quo, rather than in relation to women's issues (MacKinnon & Miller, 1987) and as potentially dangerous in relation to wife assault.

As a family therapist, I believe that an evolving family systems approach to wife battering can offer valuable theoretical perspectives and clinical interventions to address male violence against women in the family. As a feminist, I believe that the implications of certain tenets of systemic thinking must be reconsidered in order to delete gender bias and to provide a social context larger than the family in which to view the problem. The current models of intervention are attempting to expand systemic thinking so that women are not blamed for their victimization.

This chapter discusses central issues of systemic thinking in relation to wife battering, presents a rationale for a systemic approach, describes current interventive models, and offers some critical comments on the appropriateness of these models.

For the purpose of this discussion, marital/family therapy will be defined as a form of treatment based on a systems theory approach. This approach views relationships as consisting of stable sets of interacting patterns that comprise a system. Because it is patterns of interaction that are analyzed, focus shifts from isolated behaviors of individuals to a consideration of interaction. Behavior is therefore viewed as reciprocal and all members of the system are implicated in the maintenance of the behavior (Giles-Sims, 1983). Therapy is addressed to all members of the system, but they need not all be present at all times. In cases of wife abuse, marital/family therapy usually refers to the spousal system although some models include the children at some point in the treatment process.

RATIONALE FOR THE MODEL

In reviewing the literature that defines wife assault in systemic terms, the following characteristics of violent relationships give credence to a systemic analysis: (a) violence follows a cyclical pattern and is highly resistant to change unless interrupted somehow by treatment or circumstances (Cook & Frantz-Cook, 1984); (b) wife battering is the product of an interactional context characterized by repetitive sequences of transactional behavior; (c) wife battering occurs in marital systems characterized by certain relationship structures; (d) violence may serve a functional role in the maintenance of the marital system (Bograd, 1984); and (e) bringing about significant change in the use of violence as a regulatory mechanism requires not only work on controlling individual behavior, but also interventions that will help to break the homeostatic cycle that maintains the violence (Cook & Frantz-Cook, 1984).

When the violent relationship is described in these terms and the woman chooses to remain in the relationship, a rationale for family therapy exists. Even if the woman's choice to stay is an uninformed one, based on sex-role stereotyping and other gender related issues, the woman's right to her choice needs to be respected. Attempts to rescue her only render her more helpless. Assuming that there is no bias on the part of the therapist to preserve family structures, family therapy does not have the continuance of the marriage as a goal and can help the woman to make a decision to leave. A family therapy approach does not necessarily imply that family members are always seen together. Individual work with both partners can be undertaken and issues such as the safety of the woman and the man's commitment to end the violence can be addressed in individual sessions. In conjoint sessions, the couple has the opportunity to deal with the marital issues that lead to conflict and violence.

HOW FAMILY THERAPY THEORY EXPLAINS VIOLENCE AGAINST WOMEN

The major family therapy literature has not specifically addressed male violence against women in the family (Bograd, 1984). What is appearing in the literature are articles that describe characteristics of violence prone relationships, subject these relationships to a systemic analysis, and suggest a treatment plan based on these formulations (Bagarozzi & Giddings, 1983; Cook & Frantz-Cook, 1984; Margolin, 1979; Weitzman & Dreen, 1982). Violence may be described as one of many symptoms in a troubled marital system, as a sign of more underlying and more primary systemic dysfunction (e.g., structural rigidity, diffuse boundaries, or as a homeostatic mechanism maintaining the equilibrium of the system; Bograd, 1984). As an explanation of a recurring interaction in a relationship, systemic formulations help explain the chronicity and repetitiveness of battering sequences.

Weitzman and Dreen (1982) describe battering couples as locked into a complementary system in which there is rigid unilateral control with little room for negotiation. If this system remains unchallenged, violence can be avoided. However, any move toward a more symmetrical relationship threatens the homeostasis and violence erupts to re-establish complementarity. When a couple is locked into a rigid complementary system and the man has learned to be violent in response to stress, battering is likely to become the couple's resolution of conflict. Violence erupts as the couple struggles for control over the functional rules of the relationship rather than the specific problems in the relationship.

Central to the thinking of systemic theorists is the notion of circular causality. This notion attributes equal responsibility to the woman for the violence. In an effort to avoid victim blaming, Hanks and Rosenbaum (1977), in a study of women who lived with alcoholic and violent men, concluded:

> The violence that occurred between these couples cannot be simplistically explained away by either psychological theories of sadomasochistic behavior or social theories of male dominance–female submission. Certainly the women were not the reason the men became violent; the men had equally complex familial and psychological histories and, most often, a propensity to violence prior to coupling with the women. However, although not the cause, the manner in which the women often unwittingly interacted with the men during certain vulnerable times did help ignite the violence. (p. 306)

Margolin (1979) stated that each partner must accept responsibility for any actions that accelerate the abuse and that the violence should be seen as a mutual problem rather than the fault of one partner. Recent formulations addressing this dilemma conclude that the feminist view that the man is fully responsible for the battering and the systemic view that the couple are locked into a recurrent vicious cycle that is mutually maintained are not mutually exclusive. These formulations view violence as having a special nature in a relationship and therefore equal ownership of its origins is not inevitable (Cook & Frantz-Cook, 1984). This view places responsibility for violent behavior on the man but sees the maintenance of the interaction that supports violence as a shared responsibility. This thinking has important implications for treatment and seems to be the backbone on which most current systemic models addressing violence are based (Bagarozzi & Giddings, 1983; Cook & Frantz-Cook, 1984; Taylor, 1984). In order to circumvent the problems raised by circular thinking, violence is given a special status and treated independently as a primary problem.

In explaining male violence against women in the family, the family systems approach has been criticized for isolating the family from its social context. Social, political, and economic factors and the effects these forces have on family functioning and on the existence of violence in the family are ignored. Although this criticism has validity, there is an attempt to incorporate a social analysis into systemic thinking. In describing the creation of a violence prone system, Weitzman and Dreen (1982) state:

> These systems are violence prone for two main reasons: because violence is rooted in the phenomenological system or 'assumptive world' of each spouse, through personal experience with abuse as children, through sex role conditioning that encourages exploitation, and through the endemic proportion of violence in society; in short, because violence is a learned and rewarded behavior. (p. 261)

Although sociopolitical factors are not a primary consideration, the notion that family problems can be socially determined is an evolving construct in family systems theory, particularly in face of issues such as wife abuse, child abuse, and incest. These problems cannot be attributed to interactional and purely individual causes.

Giles-Sims (1983) applied a systems theory approach to wife battering in a study of 31 battered women. She examined the question of how wife battering occurs rather than why it occurs and how wife battering becomes an ongoing pattern resistant to change. She developed a six-stage systems model of wife battering to explain the development of battering behavior. The stages examine:

1. How the family system was established to allow patterns of violence to develop.
2. The sequence of interaction around the first incident of violence.
3. The homeostatic function that stabilizes violence.
4. The point at which the situation becomes unbearable to battered women.
5. Possibility of second-order change—the shifting of the systems boundaries is considered.

6. Options for battered women—from establishing of a new, more satisfactory system to returning to the former pattern.

This model uses the conceptual tools of systems theory to show how wife battering relationships develop and perhaps change over time.

MODELS OF INTERVENTION

Treatment models vary and many family therapists do not acknowledge the special nature of violence in a relationship and do not address it directly. In his recent book, *Family Kaleidoscope* (1984), Minuchin gave an account of his work with a family in which the husband has been violent toward his wife and his daughter. The violence, per se, is not dealt with and is viewed as a dysfunctional symptom of deeper problems. Aware that this approach is controversial, he commented as follows:

> As a systemic thinker, my view is that transactions among family members follow an elliptical pattern. Any act is a midpoint—a response and a stimulus in a series of recursive loops.... If we focus on a violent act, how can we intervene. (p.174) Focusing on the male as monster makes people experience their individual separation and perpetuates defensive aggression as a response to aggression. The goal should be to explore and improve people's interdependence. (p. 175)

> This approach might be seen as a form of copping out—letting the man off the hook and dismissing his destructive behavior with a shrug. I see it as the only rational way of dealing with family violence. By now my bias should be obvious. I cannot support family maintenance when the family organization is destructive to its members. The goal then is to help the family separate. But if the family wants to continue as a family unit, and if I find this feasible, I must accept my responsibility to help the family change. (p. 177)

Other family therapists who are trying to address violence directly are modifying and expanding existing interventions to adapt a family systems approach to the needs of a specialized problem.

These models have a number of features in common. They believe that the man can learn to control his violence while the couple changes the interactional sequences that lead to violence (Bagarozzi & Giddings, 1983; Cook & Frantz-Cook, 1984; Magill & Werk, 1985; Weitzman & Dreen, 1982). They treat violence directly as a primary issue and insist on no violence as a condition of treatment. Helping the woman to modify her behavior to protect herself against an abusive partner while he is learning to control his violence does not imply that she provokes the violence or is responsible for it. Most current approaches describe different stages of therapy, with the first stage aimed at cessation of violence. Most agree that to work systemically the therapist need not see all members of the system together. Men and women are seen separately particularly in the initial stages of therapy. This is an important step that facilitates accurate reporting of the violence, checking the safety of the woman, and underlining the fact that the violence is the man's problem and must be addressed by him alone.

The treatment plan outlined by Cook and Frantz-Cook (1984) is generally representational of other programs described in the literature:

> We are proposing a plan for treating couples in which battering is either the presenting problem or is revealed at some point in therapy. The major components of the treatment model are: (1) Assessment of the Problem and History of the Relationship; (2) Protection Plan (for the Battered Spouse); (3) Agreement to be Non-Violent (for the Batterer); (4) Differentiation; (5) Identifying Triangles and Coalitions; (6) Identifying Sequences and Themes, and (7) Coaching Alternative Responses. (p. 88)

Stages 1, 2, 3, and 4 are usually carried out separately to minimize the risk of violence and ensure accuracy of reporting of information. In this model, same-sex therapists work with each individual to reduce resistance and increase the client's sense of comfort, acceptance, and empathy. Assessing the problem, and taking a history of the relationship, entails the gathering of copious data about the marriage and the violence from each spouse. When the nature of the violence in the marriage is understood, the therapists can make steps to help prevent its recurrence during treatment. The woman is helped to work out a plan to protect herself if she senses that a violent incident might occur. This plan is carefully organized, rehearsed, and must clearly be understood and possible to execute. She is given some responsibility for her safety, and is thus at least partially empowered. Because empowerment is a major goal in the treatment of battered women, this first step is very important. At the same time, the man must commit himself to nonviolence. A large part of the work in this stage is to help the man become aware of when violence is likely to erupt, and to learn different responses to conflict.

Extreme dependency, enmeshment, and lack of boundaries between partners characterize most relationships where violence exists. Although the man often presents a macho and independent facade, he is usually dependent on his wife to respond to his most basic needs, and very fearful of losing her. Differentiation as a therapeutic goal begins early and aims at helping the couple to develop a capacity for separateness. A group experience for one or both partners, attending a class, seeing friends, and shopping alone, are some of the tasks aimed at individuation. These tasks should be carefully planned so that the couple can tolerate the separation and achieve success.

These first steps are common to most of the developing models and are basically aimed at stopping the violence and creating some stability in the relationship. Later stages of therapy deal with marital issues that are characterized in various ways depending on the point of view of the therapist and the unique history of the couple. Cook and Frantz-Cook (1984) work with triangles and coalitions, which involve assessing relationships with the couple's family of origin. They try to ascertain whether spouses are vulnerable to pressure from parents who bring conflict into the marital relationship thus creating triangles (e.g., wife, husband, her mother) and cross-generational coalitions. Their contention is that many of the spouses in violent relationships have not succeeded in separating from their parents. The parents have, either literally or figuratively, a strong influence on the marriage, often detrimental in nature. Identifying sequences and themes, a process that continues throughout treatment, examines the purpose the violence has served in the relationship. "The therapist hypothesizes what function it has helped maintain and what circular interaction forms a typical pattern" (Cook & Frantz-Cook, 1984, p. 90). Understanding the marital themes (e.g., distance, intimacy, control) that lead to violent episodes is important to intervention.

Weitzman and Dreen (1982) propose the following ongoing treatment plan:

1. Define thematic conflicts through a careful assessment of incidents that bring the couples into therapy.
2. Establish the point at which the complementary status shifts to symmetry and exposes the system's characteristics of volatility, rigidity, intolerance for change, and inadequacy of coping mechanisms.
3. Point out interactional sequences, formulate responses that are different than those that increase conflict. Work is done in the context of a verbal commitment from the couple to stop violence.

Bagarozzi and Giddings (1983) suggest techniques designed to keep voluntary violent couples in treatment. Because a direct attack on the couple's belief system about violence might terminate treatment, they advocate Minuchin's joining techniques to enable the therapist to communicate empathic understanding of how the spouses view themselves and their relationship. After one has gained entry into the spousal system, the therapist can begin to challenge belief systems. This approach allows the therapist to work with the couple beyond the initial resistance and move them toward a new understanding of the violence in their relationship. They state that it may be strategically wise for the therapist to:

1. Verbalize acceptance of clients' viewpoints concerning the nature of aggression to reduce initial resistance and gain entry into the system.
2. Indicate that even though aggression, as the couple defines it, may be normal, it is not acceptable.
3. Permit spouse temporary and controlled sublimation of pent up aggression only in the presence of the therapist.
4. Teach them nonviolent ways to solve differences and conflicts.

Thus, what has evolved and is still in the process of evolving, are models of intervention based on systemic principles that treat the violence as a separate and primary issue and then treat the relationship structure and rules. Causality and reciprocity are addressed by seeing the violence as a learned response to conflict by the man, which once introduced into the marital system, becomes part of the interactional sequence of the couple.

CONTENDING BELIEFS re APPROPRIATENESS
OF FAMILY THERAPY

I have already raised some of the major critical issues that question the validity of a family systems approach when dealing with wife abuse. The first criticism is that a systems perspective of families does not sufficiently take into account the social, political and economic forces that are part of the families' distresses (Bograd, 1984; Taggart, 1985). Family therapy is seen as a conservative therapy, designed to support the prevailing social order, inhibit social change, avoid the disease of society as a whole by pathologizing the individual. When applied to a problem such as violence that is so rooted in the patriarchal structure of our society, family systems theory runs the risk of pathologizing women by ignoring the socially sanctioned power imbalance between men and women.

Wilden (1972), in a critique of systemic thinking, stated that women's struggles against male dominance or privilege is termed *symmetrical*. Relationships of dominance and subservience between unequal partners are then described as competitive relations between free and legal, psychological and socioeconomic subjects. Concepts of circular causality and behavioral reciprocity implicate the woman in the causation and maintenance of the violence. But many family theorists have modified this thinking in recent years. Partners are not thought of as mutually and equally responsible for creating and maintaining the violence. Strong efforts are made to avoid blaming the victim and to assigning responsibility for battering to the man. Equal responsibility for the violence is not a concept that appears in current thinking. Most treatment approaches now single out the violence as a dangerous reality, not just another symptom, and provide ways of safeguarding the woman against the man's violence. Commitment to nonviolence by the man is an essential part of most treatment plans (Bagarozzi & Giddings, 1983; Cook & Frantz-Cook, 1984; Taylor, 1984).

In my opinion, family systems approaches are developing an evolving and valid response to the problem of wife abuse. When faced with the complexity of the relationships of violent couples, the profound attachment of the partners and the repetitive nature of the interaction; it is important to consider interactional aspects. As long as women remain committed to violent men, efforts to intervene at the couple and family level are necessary. We must respect a woman's wish to try and preserve the marriage. Models that are currently being developed stress the special nature of violence and treat it separately. Concern for the woman's safety is a primary concern. Therapists see partners individually, in groups, as well as conjointly. Thus, women have the opportunity to report honestly on the situation and to evaluate the marriage without the husband's presence. They can work on their own individual issues, such as attachment to an abusive partner, and deal with marital issues as well. This flexibility offers the opportunity to become more informed, more powerful, and more able to make a real choice about the future. Family therapy is not the treatment of choice for every violent relationship. Careful assessment is necessary to determine which couples can best respond to this approach. But it does have a role in helping to ameliorate male violence against women in the family, and systemic thinkers are struggling to adapt the theory to this serious problem.

5

Effective Interventions With Assaultive Husbands

Sally E. Palmer
Ralph A. Brown
McMaster University

PREVALENCE OF ASSAULT BY HUSBANDS

The importance of intervention with assaultive husbands has become widely accepted in North America in the 1980s. In this chapter, the term *assaultive husbands* refers to men living in a domestic relationship with a woman, whether married or not, and the term *wives* refers to the men's partners. Attention has been drawn to the widespread prevalence of domestic violence in Canada with the development of shelters for abused wives; the number of shelters tripled between 1982 and 1987, when 264 were reported (MacLeod, 1987). The provision of shelters, however, does not solve the abuse problem: The evidence indicates that 40%–69% of North American women who seek refuge in shelters eventually return to the assaultive relationship (Gondolf, 1987). It may also be expected that abusive men who are left alone will continue their behavior with new partners. Thus, there is a continuing need to assess the extent of wife abuse and to treat assaultive husbands to eliminate their violent behaviors.

In Canada, there have been no national surveys to measure directly the extent of assault by husbands. It has been estimated that close to 1 million Canadian women may be victims of marital violence by combining 1985 data from the following sources: the number of women who came to 110 shelters across Canada; the proportions seeking nonresidential help as opposed to shelters in a community study (London, Ontario); and a conservative guesstimate that one-third of those who were beaten would not seek help (MacLeod, 1987). In another Canadian study, it was conservatively estimated that 1,500 women per year in the Hamilton-

Wentworth region (population about 500,000) seek help for violence-related problems through police, the Unified Family Court, Family Services, or one of three women's shelters (Byles, 1982).

A Canadian study surveying treatment programs for assaultive husbands concluded from the literature that severe violence, such as punching or kicking, is likely to occur in about 10% of marriages, whereas less severe violence, such as pushing and slapping, is much more common (Browning, 1984). It is sometimes alleged that violence is initiated by women in a significant number of relationships, but this is not supported by evidence. The Browning survey indicated that in 95% of marital violence resulting in injury, the wife is the victim. The same figure was found in a study of domestic dispute responses by Hamilton-Wentworth regional police, 95% of the victims were women (Byles, 1980).

More direct measures of wife assault have been attempted in the United States. In a national family violence survey, based on interviews with 960 men and 1,183 women, almost one-eighth reported that they had experienced an act of violence in the marriage from which serious injuries resulted (Straus, Gelles, & Steinmetz, 1980). It has been noted by several authors that estimates of assault by husbands are conservative and tend to underestimate the true extent of the problem (Gondolf, 1985a; Straus et al., 1980; MacLeod, 1980). It is thought that women may underreport abuse by husbands because of the "insensitive response from law enforcement agencies" (Gondolf, 1985a, p. 4). In Canada, we have begun to address this issue by a nationwide policy beginning in 1986, encouraging police to lay charges against assaultive husbands (MacLeod, 1987).

It is clear from the previous discussion that marital violence is now recognized as a part of daily life for many Canadian families and that most of the victims are women. Researchers and treatment staff estimate there are many more assaulted wives who do not seek help. In the past, they have not received much support from our law enforcement system, but this has begun to change.

PAST INATTENTION TO ASSAULT BY HUSBANDS
AS AN AREA OF STUDY

There was very little research on assaultive husbands and their treatment prior to 1980, probably because wife assault was not widely identified as a social problem. It is relevant that spouse abuse, as a specific category in the Social Science Index, did not appear until 1972. Research of such taboo topics tends to be inhibited by a number of influences. Specifically, it may be difficult to identify the target population, to find subjects willing to talk about the problem, and to ensure that the reported information is generalizable. The development of both shelters for victims and treatment programs for assaultive husbands has facilitated the study of a problem that for many years remained hidden within the family.

Explanations for Assault by Husbands

Several theories or perspectives have been used to understand assault by husbands and to develop a framework for treatment. These can be categorized as psychological/clinical, structural/feminist, and social learning theories.

Psychological/Clinical Theory. This theory views the causes of assault by husbands as residing within the individual or in the couple's relationship, with some recognition given to the influence of external stress. From this perspective, treatment is directed toward improving communication between the spouses. Some earlier studies suggested that the male's presumed individual psychopathology was the main contributing variable to assault by husbands, for example his sociopathic and impulsive nature, his authoritarian and patriarchal characteristics, and his low self-esteem (Martin, 1976; Pagelow, 1981). Abusive husbands are described as prone to temper tantrums; insecure (i.e., needing to keep the environment stable and nonthreatening); jealous and possessive; and subject to alcohol abuse (Walker, 1983). These attempts to explain violence as an outcome of individual psychopathology seem insufficient, as most assaultive husbands are not considered to be psychiatrically or even psychologically disturbed. In the authors' experiences with men in treatment, to be described later, they are usually functioning, accepted members of the community.

In addition to the aforementioned interpersonal characteristics, the psychological/clinical approach recognizes the role of interactional variables, such as poor marital relationships and external stress. Specifically, economic stress related to low income, unemployment, and part-time work have all been associated with violence in male partners (Roberts, 1987; Straus et al., 1980). Unemployed men are twice as likely as full-time employed men to severely abuse their wives. An even greater discrepancy is reported for men employed part time: They abuse their wives three times more often than full-time employed men (Straus et al., 1980). It is also suggested that tension at work is associated with wife assault. As with theories of individual pathology, the concept of stress-related violence does not account for the variability among men subjected to similar stresses. Many men experience economic stress, yet do not resort to violence.

Another form of stress offered as an explanation of family violence is that experienced with the addition of children to a family. One study indicated that violence rarely occurred in families with no children, whereas it was found increasingly as the number of children increased to six (Straus et al., 1980).

In summary, traditional psychological/clinical theories tend to focus on deterministic explanations for wife assault, based on individual pathology, sometimes giving recognition to the interaction between personality and external stress. These explanations fail to take account of the social environment in which wife abuse occurs; also they seem to absolve assaultive men from responsibility for their behavior. These societal and responsibility issues are analyzed by the other two theoretical approaches.

Structural/Feminist Theory. This theory tends to view wife assault as rooted in the patriarchal structures of society, specifically in the traditional view that husbands should wield the balance of power in families. Assault by husbands has been found to be more prevalent where power in the relationship resides with the husband; it is suggested that "violence is used by the most powerful family member as a means of legitimizing his or her dominant position" (Straus et al., 1980, p. 193). From this perspective, an argument can be made that men with low socioeconomic status are more likely to resort to family violence: Society accords them the balance of power over family decision making, yet they lack resources such as knowledge, education, prestige, and income that would legitimize their positions. Consequently, these men may attempt to secure their power position at the only level where they feel superior (i.e., a physical expression of strength). From this viewpoint, spousal abuse can be seen as reflecting the results of unequal distribution of power in the wider society: The man is penalized by social disadvantage outside the family and passes on the penalty to the weaker members of his family.

The feminist analysis also notes that our society accepts violence as a means of resolving conflict. It has been noted that public and professionals alike express ambivalence about the normative boundaries of violence, especially at the less severe end of the spectrum (Finkelhor, 1983). In the United States, a national survey found that 31.3% of the men and 24.6% of the women viewed physical means of expression (e.g., slapping) as a normal aspect of the marriage relationship (Straus et al., 1980). These findings led the researchers to coin the phrase "the marriage license is a hitting license" (p.48).

The view that some wife abuse is normal is also implied in the clinical explanation, just given, that violence is stress related. The idea that men experiencing tension at work may return home and abuse their wives implies that violence inflicted upon wives is an understandable reaction, perhaps a preferred alternative, to open expression of frustration in the workplace. Another explanation (Straus et al., 1980) pointed out that "a man who feels threatened and devalued at work may use force and violence in his home to restore his sense of being master of his life. Only a cog in a machine at work, a man can still be lord of the manor when he returns home" (p. 188). The feminist perspective rejects explanations based on individual personality or stress as inadequate. Instead, it focuses on the extent to which assault by husbands is encouraged by gender inequalities that place women in subordinate roles (Fagan, Stewart, & Hansen, 1983).

Feminist theory also addresses the popular perception that assaulted wives have provoked their husband's violence or that they are content with the status quo; this perception is cited as an example of blaming the victim. The structural/feminist approach takes the view that family violence is never justified as a response to provocation. Regarding the tendency of women to stay with or return to assaultive men, there are strong economic and safety reasons for this. Economically, it is well recognized that single mothers with children are at high risk of living in poverty. As for safety, the Canadian media are continually reporting examples of men abusing or murdering women who have left them; from the authors' experience in Hamilton-Wentworth, many women seeking help receive threats of revenge from their husbands if they do not return home.

The structural/feminist perspective explains wife abuse in terms of unequal power accorded by society to men and women. This is reflected in social acceptance of traditional marriage roles, and in ambivalent social attitudes toward less severe forms of physical aggression, including blaming the victim for generating or tolerating violence. Social class inequalities are also identified as interacting with the husband's power-seeking behavior as expressed in wife assault. Structural/feminist theory goes beyond the psychological/clinical approach in examining the behavior of assaultive husbands as a social, rather than a private problem. It introduces the aspect of social justice, by examining marital violence in terms of power inequities and the implications for harm to weaker members of society, both women and children.

Social Learning Theory. The third theory explains the behavior of assaultive husbands in terms of modeling and imitation (Bandura, 1973, 1977). There is ample documentation of assaultive husbands having learned to use violence through observation in their families and other socializing experiences.

Reports by female victims of their male partners' histories showed numerous precedents for violent behavior in the men's histories: These included childhood experiences of family violence, their own violent behavior as children (toward people and pets), and later criminality as well as military experience (Walker, 1983). Social learning has also been observed by therapists who work with children from violent families. These children have learned from observing parental arguments that physical violence is effective in reinforcing their father's power (Pressman, 1984). It has been suggested that children witnessing their parents' violence are likely to learn the following lessons: hitting is normal behavior in intimate relationships; it is an effective means of influencing others within the family; and it is morally acceptable to use force as a last resort (Straus et al., 1980). Researchers have compared men who had witnessed marital violence as children to those from nonviolent homes, and found that the former group assaulted their wives almost three times as often (Straus et al., 1980). The difference increased when only the men from the most violent 20% of families were considered: These men had a rate of wife beating 10 times greater than the sons of nonviolent parents.

As well as learning from observations of parents' interaction, children are socialized to sex roles by family, school, and community. In our society, this involves different expectations regarding aggression for males and females. The socialization of girls tends to emphasize social skills, whereas boys are often reinforced for competitive and aggressive behavior. From this viewpoint, it is understandable that males who witness family violence between their parents will carry this into their own marriages, and that their wives will not be equipped to cope with it.

In summary, there is considerable evidence to support a social learning perspective on wife assault, in terms of repetition of family behavior by the next generation, and differential socialization of males and females. Once accepted, the social learning model becomes a useful framework for treatment, as it implies that men from violent homes can unlearn their abusive behavior. When compared to psychological/clinical theories that view behavior as predetermined by indelible early experiences, social learning provides more impetus for change.

Each of the three theoretical perspectives examined here makes a contribution toward an integrated understanding of the etiology and dynamics of wife abuse. In our view, psychological/clinical theories are useful at an individual level, and generate ideas for treatment, but they have several limitations. They support a deterministic view of behavior, the issue of responsibility is not addressed, and little attention is given to the social environment that facilitates husbands' aggression against their wives. Structural/feminist theory is not oriented to the treatment of assaultive husbands, but it contributes to a framework in which treatment can take place. Specifically, it highlights the social norms and institutions that lead to and reinforce marital violence, and holds out a goal of gender equality and social justice. Finally, social learning theory contributes a view of abusive behavior as learned through socialization, including experience in the family of origin as learned behavior. This points to the possibility that such behavior may be unlearned through a corrective socialization experience.

THEORETICAL PERSPECTIVES
AS A BASIS FOR TREATMENT

Based on the previous discussion, our preference is for an integrated approach to treating assaultive husbands, including all three perspectives, with emphasis on social learning as providing the most direction for treatment. In practice, the scope of the social learning approach can be very broad. It can include educating assaultive husbands to understand family violence, to accept the long-term advantages of democratic power sharing within in the family, and to learn nonviolent ways of solving problems. This education can be done at a personal level, by helping men to consider the unwanted consequences of their habitual behavior, as well as a philosophical level, using the structural/feminist analysis to appeal to their sense of social justice.

Psychological/clinical theory is also useful in helping assaultive husbands to cue in to the emotions and stresses that precede their outbreaks of violence. They need to recognize and discuss feelings of frustration and helplessness, if they are to gain control over their aggressive behavior. Most Canadian treatment programs currently in operation tend to be eclectic, incorporating some aspects from each of the above perspectives (Browning, 1984). The remainder of this chapter describes the most favored approach to treatment and the existing research on its effectiveness. It also examines impediments to treatment, as well as difficulties in evaluating outcomes. Specific attention is given to the Hamilton-Wentworth Family Violence Treatment Program and its evaluation component, which will reach completion in late 1989.

Treatment for Assaultive Husbands

Predominance of Group Treatment

The format for treatment ranges from individual or couple counseling, through professionally led groups for men alone and for couples, to self-help groups. As the literature indicates, however, there is a definite preference for group counseling (Sinclair, 1985). Professionals who have tried alternative approaches with assaultive husbands report better progress with groups (Ganley, 1981) and the authors could find no reports contradicting this. Most groups are men only; in fact it has been suggested that couples' groups are contraindicated until the violence is under control. When a wife discusses her husband's assaultive behavior in a couples' group, she risks his anger and possible backlash for exposing him (Bograd, 1984; Star, 1983). As the evidence so clearly favors the group approach, the discussion here is limited to this model.

Group treatment is expected to have both direct and indirect benefits for assaultive husbands. Direct benefits include the ability of other group members to confront men's denials and to support intended or accomplished behavioral change (Ganley, 1981). Groups are also recommended as promoting interpersonal skills and emotive communication (Purdy & Nickle, 1981) and as lessening the low self-esteem thought to contribute to abuse (Brownell & Shumaker, 1985).

The indirect benefits of group treatment include the opportunity for men to develop new relationships to offset their excessive emotional dependency on their female partners (Adams, 1981; Ganley, 1981). This is particularly true in self-help groups, where a support network can be developed that functions outside group meetings. Through the group experience, men learn how to ask for help from others; they are also encouraged to take a nurturing role by offering support to other group members, which may be a new experience for them (Pressman, 1984). The value of group support has been cited by men who successfully gave up violence after a group treatment experience: They said the group offered them acceptance and firm direction, thus enabling them to change their behavior as well as enhancing their self esteem (Gondolf & Hanneken, 1987).

Within the group format, a variety of methods has been used with assaultive husbands. These include education, behavior modification, insight-oriented therapy and catharsis. They are usually combined, as wife assault is a complex phenomenon requiring more than one approach (Steinfeld, 1986).

At last report, there were 44 groups for abusive husbands operating in Canada including 19 in Ontario and every province except Newfoundland (Health and

Welfare Canada, 1986). Canadian treatment groups appear to have common basic assumptions and principles. They are similar to U.S. treatment programs that have been described in the literature (EMERGE, 1981; Ganley, 1981; Purdy & Nickle, 1981). This similarity probably reflects the rapid growth in interest and financial support for programs addressing wife abuse since 1980; most people involved in initiating programs have had access to an information network and have been able to build on the experience of others.

Basic Assumptions in Treatment

The following assumptions seem to be characteristic of most Canadian treatment programs for assaultive husbands (Browning, 1984; Sinclair, 1985). Some of these basic assumptions are drawn from the structural/feminist model. For example, it is explicitly acknowledged that there is a power differential between husbands and wives, and that our society has tended to tolerate less severe forms of physical aggression by husbands. In order to counter this, group leaders place the responsibility for violent behavior squarely on the offender. Attempts by the men to excuse their violent behavior because of provocation are not accepted on the basis that aggression is never justified.

Social learning theory is also a part of the basic framework as group leaders tend to discuss the men's use of aggression in terms of learned behavior, and state clearly their goal of having participants unlearn this means of problem solving. It is also made explicit that the dominant culture supports male violence as a problem-solving method, and that assaultive husbands must alter their attitudes if any behavioral change is to be lasting. Assumptions from clinical theory are probably less explicit, but it is recognized that husbands may be strongly attached to their aggressive behavior; they are reluctant to relinquish its rewards such as the release of pent-up feelings and reaffirmation of their control over their wives. From this assumption, it is clear that the men's motivation must be strong and they must feel there is some compensation for giving up the immediate rewards of violence.

Principles for Treatment

Group leaders working with assaultive husbands usually adhere to principles such as concern for the safety of both partners, a value-free attitude toward offenders, and emphasis on engagement techniques to overcome the offenders' initial denial and resistance to treatment (Pressman, 1984; Sinclair, 1985). To ensure the safety of both victim and offender, the victim is invited to come for at least one interview; if possible, she is involved in a group or in ongoing counseling.

A value-free attitude by the leader means accepting the offender as a whole person with strengths as well as weaknesses. This facilitates the relationship with the offender as well as with the victim; the latter often has genuine concern for her partner and would be alienated by a judgmental approach. A value-free attitude also helps leaders to accept the behavior of victims, who may return to an abusive relationship or swing ambivalently between separation and reunion.

Engagement of the offender was identified as a major problem in a survey of 44 U.S. programs (Roberts, 1984). The leader begins with identifying and responding to realistic expectations about treatment and dispelling those that are unrealistic, such as the leader's ability to effect reconciliation with a departed partner. At the same time, the leader offers hope and establishes credibility by describing positive results achieved with others like the offender.

Engagement also includes orienting members to the goals and content of group treatment in order to enhance their level of comfort and willingness to participate. They should be introduced to the major themes on which the group is likely to focus: the consequences of violent behavior, particularly loss of the partner; alternative coping strategies, and the offenders' feelings about their own violent behavior.

After initial engagement, the offender may need help to maintain his commitment to treatment. The source of referral can often reinforce continuing participation. Probation officers are the most obvious reinforcers, as they have mandated power. Other referral sources include lawyers, family physicians, psychiatrists, organizations/institutions providing physical or mental health services, government and voluntary social services agencies, professionals in private practice, and other community sources such as church, school, employer, friends, and relatives. Nonprofessional referral sources must be used with discretion, but some outside reinforcement of treatment-seeking is important when participation falters.

In summary, group leaders are generally committed to the goal of a nonviolent family environment; they adopt a nonjudgmental attitude toward both partners; and they give much attention to the offenders' initial engagement, as well as reinforcing their ongoing participation in treatment.

Preference for Court-Mandated Treatment

Many professionals reporting in the literature prefer court-mandated to voluntary subjects (Ganley, 1981; Pressman, 1984), although this is not unanimous. A survey of 44 program administrators showed mixed views on the issue (Roberts, 1984). Court support for treatment counters the perception of offenders that society will tolerate domestic violence.

A court order also provides the needed motivation for assaultive husbands to seek help and change their behavior, ensuring that they cannot easily drop out on impulse. The drop-out rates in group treatment are high: One survey indicated that one third to one half of men dropped out after the first session (Feazell, Mayers, & Deschner, 1984). Withdrawal is understandable, because the expectation for change is likely to threaten the beliefs and and coping methods of already insecure men. Attendance tends to be better in programs with a higher percentage of court-mandated referrals (Roberts, 1984).

Another benefit of court involvement is the length of time required for effective treatment. Because violence is difficult to relinquish, offenders need external motivation until treatment helps them develop internal controls. It has been suggested that a 1 year follow-up is necessary to ensure the offender can maintain the skills needed for anger control (Pressman, 1984). Court-ordered treatment usually includes a probation period, during which offenders can easily be returned to court if the violence recurs.

In summary, court-mandated referrals are useful in ensuring participation in treatment. The experience with the court process and fear of recurrence probably provides good motivation for the men to change their behavior and, concurrently, their attitudes about the use of aggression.

Hamilton-Wentworth Family Violence Treatment Program

The preference for court-mandated referrals to treatment, will be tested out by the Hamilton-Wentworth Family Violence Treatment Program (H-W FVTP): outcomes for court-mandated subjects are compared with those for volunteers. The program follows the basic assumptions and principles outlined here; its specific goals and details of implementation are described next, for the benefit of readers who are relatively unfamiliar with such programs.

Format. The Hamilton-Wentworth program differs from most men's treatment groups in attempting to engage the abused partners in concurrent women's groups. The format is family focused, with the intention of addressing the power imbalance from both sides (i.e., helping women to unlearn traditional attitudes toward male dominance, and to learn better methods of protecting themselves from abuse). Only 25% of the victims have been willing to join a group since evaluation of the groups began in February 1987, and these families will be compared to the others to explore whether this family focus is associated with better outcomes as hypothesized. The following discussion covers only the men's groups, as treatment for husbands is the focus of this chapter.

Goals. The program goals follow the assumptions and principles previously set out. In keeping with social learning theory, one goal is to have men examine the nature of domestic violence in their marriages: their use of aggression, and its short- and long-term consequences. The outcome goal of this process is to have the men accept that violence is unacceptable and that power should be democratically distributed in the family.

Another goal is to elicit the men's emotions (i.e., how they feel leading up to the violence, immediately after it erupts, and after the urgency has subsided). One outcome goal of this process is to have men gain cognitive, then behavioral, control of their emotions so they can preempt the eruption of violence. Catharsis in the group may also help to drain off men's self-anger, which might otherwise be transformed into reduced self-esteem; as noted earlier, low self-esteem is a common element in men who bully their wives.

Another outcome goal is to have men recognize the nature of the short-term emotional gains that make violence hard to give up. Finally, contemplation of the guilt or remorse they feel after the event can be used as a motivator to give up abusive behavior. Sometimes men's preoccupation with guilt becomes immobilizing; sharing of feelings in the group may help to resolve these feelings to the point where the energy invested can be freed up for constructive change.

Content. The goals listed here are achieved through a program that combines information giving, discussion of attitudes and feelings, and teaching of skills for dealing with anger and frustration. The *information* provided to the men's groups includes the legal, social, and emotional issues related to domestic violence; historical perspective and myths; as well as the nature and causes of violence.

The *discussion topics* include confrontation with men's denial of responsibility for violence. Denial is treated by asserting the man's responsibility for deciding to use violence, no matter what the provocation and how great his anger or frustration. Other discussion topics include the benefits of stopping the violence; the self-image of offenders, their values, and life goals, as well as experience with personal change during the treatment period.

The content includes teaching *skills* to deal with feelings and behavior includes recognizing cues to violence; finding other behavioral options; techniques to cope with stress and manage anger, such as relaxation, cueing, and self-talk; and communicating more effectively on a verbal level. The latter skill is important, because many violent men experience a sense of helplessness in conflicts with their wives whom, they feel, can express themselves more effectively. As noted by Pressman (1984), they often deal with their helplessness by "blaming, not listening, name-calling, interrupting, defensiveness..." (p. 66), so it is helpful for the group to practice active listening, expressing hurt feelings directly, and checking out assumptions about what has been said.

Impediments to Providing Effective Service

Professionals working with violent men report a number of impediments to treatment. Initially, these men tend to deny the importance of the violence, or rationalize that their wives provoked them, rather than accepting responsibility for their behavior. At this stage, they are unwilling to engage in self-examination. Another impediment is that many wife abusers have little insight into their own feelings, having habitually acted these out rather than allowing themselves to experience them.

In keeping with their defensiveness, assaultive husbands are inclined to be hypersensitive to criticism, so they overreact to any comment that could be interpreted as a negative judgment on their behavior. In addition, many of these men use aggression when threatened, so they may attempt to intimidate the leader or other group members. The group leader's role is to label any attempts to control the group by intimidation, and to encourage group members to express their reactions to the aggressive member. Such discussion can heighten members' insight into how they use and react to intimidation generally, and in their marriages in particular.

Men who have been violent outside the home or who have criminal records are especially likely to challenge the leader's authority, to resist the group process or drop out of treatment. This is even more reason to label and discuss aggressive or intimidating behavior when it occurs in the group. As for drop-outs, with men who are court mandated, the leader must be prepared to invoke the judicial system to keep them involved.

In summary, most treatment for assaultive husbands in Canada tends to be in a group format; there are basic assumptions and principles that are widely held among therapists and these tend to determine the group goals and content. Experience with wife abusers has shown they are difficult to treat but some of the difficulties are addressed by using the group method. Next, we examine the available information about the effectiveness of treatment for assaultive husbands.

Efficacy of Treatment

There has been little substantial evaluation of different treatment modalities with assaultive husbands (Gondolf, 1987). Group programs have received the most attention, but the evaluation research tends to be inconclusive, either because of reliance on self-reports from the subjects or the treatment staff or the absence of a valid comparison group. Treatment subjects tend to be compared with men who apply for treatment but do not follow through, or those who drop out during the treatment period. Finally, the published evaluations have not given attention to the group process itself, so there is little empirical evidence to support the preference for group treatment (Gondolf, 1987).

Measures of success tend to be of two kinds: before–after scores on personality tests; and estimates of violent behavior after treatment. The following three studies reported posttreatment improvement in personality or interpersonal characteristics. Ninety-two men, after 20 group sessions, showed significant change in the desired direction on scales of extreme forms of anger toward partners, anger toward work/friend relationships, depression, attitudes toward women, and jealousy (Saunders & Hanusa, 1986). Similarly, 24 men receiving group psychotherapy for 6 months showed significant change in the hypothesized direction on child abuse potential, depression, psychopathic deviation, global distress, effective communication, and problem-solving communication (Myers, 1984). The third study cited improvement after counseling on standard measures of marital satisfaction, communication skills, and self-esteem (Neidig & Friedman, 1984). These studies measured only short-term gains, but the results do suggest that treatment may improve offenders' communication skills, their attitudes toward women and toward themselves (the latter point is indicated by higher self-esteem and less depression).

Studies measuring post-treatment violence report fairly high success rates. A national survey indicated that 66%–75% of those who completed a prescribed program were nonviolent after 1 year according to self- or staff reports (Gondolf, 1987; Feazell, Mayers, & Deschner, 1984). A comparative follow-up 6 months after treatment found that 61% ($N = 31$) of men completing at least half the program reported nonviolence, whereas men who contacted the program but did not enroll ($N = 23$) were estimated to be twice as violent (Gondolf, 1987). These studies have the weakness related to self-reports—the tendency for men to underreport their violence. Also, the comparison in the latter study is questionable: The treatment group may be expected to be more motivated than those who failed to enroll; thus they might have improved as a result of the situation creating their motivation, rather than from the treatment itself.

Another follow-up study compared program completers with noncompleters, and included verification interviews with wives. The nonviolence was similar to the studies just mentioned, with 67% of completers reported as nonviolent, compared to 54% of noncompleters, but the follow-up was shorter, at 4.5 months (Edleson & Grusznski, 1986). The tendency to underreport violence is suggested by discrepancies between the reports of offenders and victims. A study of three programs in Texas showed that 75% of the men reported nonviolence compared to 55% of their partners (Stacey & Shupe, 1984).

In summary, there are few useful evaluative studies of treatment outcomes with assaultive husbands, mainly because of subjectivity and inadequate comparison groups. Given these limitations, it does appear that treatment helps to eliminate violence in about 55%–75% of cases. As well, treatment is associated with improvement in men's communication skills, attitudes toward women, and self-concepts. In order to establish these tentative findings on a sounder basis, evaluation needs to be carried out more systematically. The group process itself needs to be given attention in terms of connecting outcomes to what happens in the group. The evaluation of the Hamilton-Wentworth program addresses both these aspects.

Evaluation of the Hamilton-Wentworth Program

The Hamilton-Wentworth Family Violence Treatment Program began in 1985 with groups for both men and women. The evaluation component began its pilot study in August 1986, and will follow its subjects for 12 months after treatment ending in 1989. From the outset, attention was given to integrating the evaluation component into the ongoing treatment program with minimal intrusion. This greatly depended on the goodwill and cooperation of the group leaders.

As mentioned earlier, the H-W FVTP differs from many others in carrying on a concurrent group for the partners of the assaultive men. The evaluation component is also unique in having a control group. It was agreed by judges hearing wife assault cases that they would sentence convicted men to probation, specifying that they should participate in the H-W FVTP. Men who were referred within 3 weeks of a new group commencing would be mandated to receive treatment; the others would be mandated to participate as controls although their probation officers could seek treatment elsewhere if deemed appropriate. Projects reported in the literature have not had control groups; they have depended on pre–postmeasures or have compared treatment subjects with men who dropped out of treatment early which does not provide a valid comparison.

The H-W FVTP treatment groups were comprised of convicted men mandated to receive treatment and men who came voluntarily. Originally it was planned to have separate treatment for the two categories of referral; but referrals from the court were sporadic, so the two were combined. Another aspect of the evaluation is monitoring of the group process by videotape for 3 of 10 sessions with each group of men and women. This will enable the study of the group process and explore potential associations between group dynamics and outcome.

Measurement

Measures are taken of the men on various dimensions at three points in time: before treatment; after the 10-week group treatment program; and 12 months later. The measures include demographic data, personality characteristics, attitudes to violence, past and present antisocial behavior (including wife assault), and other aspects of family functioning. Personality characteristics are measured by the Basic Personality Inventory (Hill & Jackson, 1984) and family functioning is measured by the Family Assessment Device (Byles, Byrne, Boyle, & Offord, 1988). Outcomes will be calculated by comparing pre- and posttreatment scores on these measures, with a 1 year follow-up. The men's partners will also be questioned about the men's continuation or cessation of abusive behavior and court records will be checked. The analysis will control for initial variation in personality, attitudes, and behavior among the three groups of men.

For the exploratory aspect of the evaluation, we have developed instruments for monitoring the subjects' behavior during the groups. The videotapes are monitored for individual behavior, both verbal and nonverbal; the group process is being evaluated in terms of participation, indigenous leadership, supportive/destructive interaction, and responses to leader's interventions. By analyzing these dimensions in relation to treatment outcomes, we hope to generate some hypotheses about group process, individual participation, and leadership in the treatment of assaultive husbands.

In summary, the H-W FVTP was developed as a family-focused approach to the treatment of wife assault, with a strong evaluative component, including a randomized control group. The evaluation will compare the outcomes of convicted offenders, after treatment and one year later, with those of similarly convicted offenders, as well as volunteers. Outcomes will also be compared for men whose abused partners receive concurrent treatment. The group process will also be studied for indications of which aspects of treatment are associated with positive outcomes.

Difficulties in Conducting Research on Spouse Abuse

Research on assaultive husbands has not kept pace with the proliferation of treatment programs. It has been suggested that the privacy and intimacy of the family as an institution makes it difficult to study family behavior accurately (Straus et al., 1980). Difficulties may also arise from the predominance of males as the offenders, as men are less likely than women to seek help or to participate in research.

A particular drawback in organizing practice-based research with assaultive husbands is the relative lack of professional networks needed to coordinate referral, treatment, and evaluation. These networks are slowly developing, according to the authors' experience in the Hamilton-Wentworth region. Compared to the problem of child abuse, however, professionals who might cooperate in research tend to be marginally involved in the movement against wife abuse (Gondolf, 1985a).

Dependence on cooperation from the criminal justice system for referrals is another issue in researching wife abuse. Treatment programs for assaultive husbands attract some voluntary clients, but the more serious cases are usually processed and referred by the court. In the Hamilton-Wentworth FVTP, a few court referrals were being made at the time the evaluation research began, but the numbers were lower than anticipated. Inquiries revealed that a number of judges felt these men could not be changed through treatment, so would not refer them to the program.

In order to generate an adequate study population, the researchers and treatment staff presented the program and its rationale at a series of meetings with key professionals in the legal system: probation officers, Crown Attorneys, defense counsels and judges in both Family and Criminal Courts. In addition to convincing them to send convicted wife abusers to the H-W FVTP, we also required their cooperation in assigning men to a probation-only comparison group. Over a 6-month period, we gradually gained the cooperation of about 50% of Criminal Court judges. The formation of the control group was the most difficult aspect: Resistance came from most of the legal professionals, as well as from treatment staff and government officials responsible for funding the treatment. These groups were oriented to providing treatment to everyone who needed it, yet the research design called for a control group whose members would ideally receive no treatment. To achieve cooperation, the research team had to modify two aspects of the design. First, arrangements were made to inform the judge, before sentencing, whether the man would be in the treatment or comparison group, so this could be made clear in his sentence. Second, it was agreed that the comparison subjects could receive individual treatment, to be arranged by their probation officers.

In summary, useful research on the treatment of spouse abuse has been slow to develop. This may be partly attributable to social attitudes, but there is a cumbersome system to be negotiated in order to recruit court-mandated offenders and particularly to collect a comparable group of subjects for comparison. It is hoped that the results of evaluating the H-W FVTP will help to fill this gap.

CONCLUSION

As this chapter has shown, the treatment of assaultive husbands has developed in North America as a response to the growing public awareness of domestic violence. Treatment programs in Canada have proliferated during the 1980s, particularly treatment groups with structured, time-limited programs. Group leaders generally adhere to common assumptions and principles, recognizing the social context of domestic violence and seeking a democratic distribution of power in both the family and the broader society. The goals and content of treatment generally emphasize a social learning approach, geared to changing men's attitudes, teaching alternatives to violence, and dealing with feelings that underlie abusive behavior.

Existing research has shown that personality change and reduction of violence are associated with group treatment, but it is not known whether these changes may result from preexisting motivation or from the treatment itself. It may be that men who begin and continue in treatment voluntarily are highly motivated by fear of losing their wives or by a desire to win back a departed wife. Men who are sent by the court may change because they want to avoid future encounters with the legal system. The control group in the H-W FVTP is expected to help separate the effects of treatment from the effects of preexisting conditions. The evaluation will also provide some beginning answers as to the comparative outcomes of treatment with voluntary and court-mandated subjects.

A particularly important aspect of the research is the exploration of the treatment process. Assuming that group treatment is found to be associated with good outcomes (i.e., the men in treatment function better and are less violent than those in the control group, there remain questions about how treatment may have facilitated these changes). We expect that our analysis of the group process and the behavior of individual men in the groups, as associated with outcome, will provide a beginning understanding of the salient aspects of treatment. By the cumulative efforts of researchers studying treatment and its effects, we should be able to build on the strengths of our existing programs and develop new approaches to treat men who have abused their wives.

ACKNOWLEDGMENTS

The authors are co-investigators for an evaluation of the Family Violence Treatment Program at Family Services of Hamilton-Wentworth. The program and evaluation were initiated by the late Jack Byles, D.S.W.; Maru Barrera, Ph.D. is a co-investigator; Susan Kalaher, B.A.& Sc. is the Research Assistant.

The evaluation project is being funded by a grant of $108,000, over three years, from the Women's Directorate of the Ontario Ministry of Community and Social Services.

6

Effects of Family Violence on Children: New Directions for Research and Intervention

Timothy E. Moore
Debra Pepler
Reet Mae
Michele Kates
York University

*F*amily violence presents a major concern to society as it places both women and children at risk for physical and mental health problems. Although considerable attention has been focused on the victims of child and wife abuse, only recently have children exposed to interparental violence also been considered as victims at risk for psychological problems. The concern is not only for their health and safety, but also for their psychological and behavioral adjustment. In addition, there is apprehension about the long-term consequences of receiving daily lessons in aggressive behavior. Children from violent homes, even though they themselves may not have been physically abused, may be viewed as at risk to perpetuate violence and abuse during adulthood. Intergenerational patterns of violence are a consistent research finding (Hughes & Hampton, 1984).

Children exposed to interparental family violence are the focus of this chapter which is organized according to some hypotheses we have made about the effects of exposure to family violence on children. We are currently examining some of the characteristics of violent families, some aspects of the child's psychological makeup, and the influence of these factors on the behavioral and psychological consequences of witnessing domestic violence. We hope to learn how the presence of certain risk factors predisposes the child to psychological and behavioral adjustment problems. We anticipate that the data we collect will permit some inferences about the psychological origins of the adjustment problems of children exposed to family violence. In what follows, some preliminary findings from this research project are used to illustrate the conceptual focus of current investigations of the consequences of interparental violence. To date we have tested 25 mothers and 32 children aged 6–12 who had recently moved to shelters because of interparental violence. Finally, we describe some current interventions as they address the apparent needs of such children and we close with a discussion of the implications of our hypotheses for future program development.

OVERVIEW OF THE RESEARCH

Behavioral and Academic Effects

Only during the last decade or so have researchers conducted specific studies of the behavioral adjustment of children of battered women. In general, it appears that both boys and girls exposed to interparental violence are at risk for internalising behavior problems (e.g., depression, anxiety, withdrawal) and social competence problems (e.g., school performance, social involvement) (Christopoulos, Cohn, Sullivan-Hanson, Kraft, & Emery, 1985). In addition, boys seem to be particularly at risk for externalizing behavior problems (such as aggressiveness, hyperactivity, and delinquency) compared to children who have not been exposed to family violence (Hughes & Barad, 1983; Jaffe, Wolfe, Wilson, & Zak, 1986b; Jouriles, Barling, & O'Leary, 1987). Further analyses of the boys' behavior problems indicated that they were characterized by inappropriate social interactions such as aggressiveness toward peers, destructiveness, mood changes and disobedience (Jaffe, Wolfe, Wilson, & Zak, 1986b).

Some investigators have suggested that the effects of witnessing parental violence may be more subtle for girls or may involve changes in thinking and social perceptions that show up later in life (Jaffe, Wolfe, Wilson, & Zak, 1985). It is also possible that the discrepant findings with respect to the effects of exposure to family violence on boys versus girls may be a result of research that has confounded sex and the witness/victim distinction. Alternatively, there may be a gender difference in the sheer amount of exposure. Hetherington, Cox, and Cox (1982) reported that parents were more likely to quarrel in front of boys than girls. If this also holds true for domestic violence, then girls and boys, even in the same family, may not be exposed to the same degree of trauma.

Sex differences notwithstanding, there is little doubt that exposure to interparental violence often has profound effects on children that are exhibited by passive, internalized behavioral responses (e.g., anxiety, depression) or active, externalized behavioral responses (e.g., hyperactivity, delinquency). The seriousness of these difficulties is evident from their similarity to those of children who have been abused (Hershorn & Rosenbaum, 1985; Wolfe & Mosk, 1983).

Although there is limited research on the academic performance of children of battered women, they were rated lower than controls on the social competence scale of the Achenbach Child Behavior Checklist (Achenbach & Edelbrock, 1983), which includes a subscale for school performance (Wolfe, Zak, Wilson, & Jaffe, 1986). Children recently exposed to family violence were reported by their mothers as having lower school performance compared to children from nonviolent families. Another indication of the potential risk of academic problems for these children comes from the research on children from separated and divorced families who reportedly experience (depending on their age) a number of academic problems. Two years following divorce, preschool children tend to do more poorly on performance IQ tasks that require attention and planful thinking compared to children from intact families (Hetherington, Cox & Cox, 1979). Older children (9–11 years) decline in their school performance during the first year following separation (Wallerstein & Kelly, 1976). For these older children, school work styles appear to be particularly affected, with the children showing deficits in preparedness, concentration, attentiveness, and task completion, compared to children from nondivorced families (Hess & Camera, 1979).

The existence of behavioral adjustment problems and academic difficulties for children of battered women is supported by our observations in the Earlcourt Reception Classroom for children of battered women at Huron Street School in Toronto. There is a wide range of behavioral responses among the children in the classroom. Some exhibit extreme internalizing adjustment problems such as anxiety, depression, somatic complaints, and bad dreams. Others, particularly boys, exhibit externalizing adjustment problems such as fighting, impulsiveness, and disobedience. Not all children, however, are so adversely affected; many seem to be able to cope with the violent family environment without major adjustment problems.

With respect to school performance, many children in the Reception Classroom are behind academically. Although some of the academic problems may be due to learning disabilities, others may simply have fallen behind due to inconsistent attendance related to family transience. The children's academic problems are often compounded by an inability to concentrate that may be attributable to anxiety, a learned response of inattention, overtiredness, illness, and/or other factors related to family crisis.

Psychological Resources

After 30 years of extensive research on the development of aggressive behavior in children, Eron (1987) concluded that "in order to predict complex human behavior like aggression, we must know ... what is going on inside the head of the subject" (p. 441). As a consequence of living in a violent family, children may exhibit relatively conspicuous behavioral adjustment problems. Other effects, however, are much more covert and have received relatively little research attention. We believe that the development of the child's thoughts, feelings, and cognitive operations are important because they mediate or underlie the adjustment problems outlined here.

Rutter (1987) has speculated on the importance of protective factors that may influence a child's response to some stressful event. Some protective factors are internal; in other words, they pertain to the psychological processes and reactions marshalled to deal with adversity, as opposed to more external resources such as the availability of a warm, caring, and supportive parent. Protective internal resources are a function of children's cognitive ideations about themselves, their experiences, and their appraisal of their own personal adequacy. Those who demonstrate resilience in adversity are more likely to have positive self-esteem, self-confidence, and a belief in their ability to deal with change.

Another type of protective factor pertains to social problem-solving skills. These include both interpersonal sensitivity and effective use of alternative methods to aggression for dealing with social conflicts. Women involved in battering situations exhibit poorer social problem-solving skills than women from nonviolent homes (Claerhout, Elder, & Janes, 1982). They produced more avoidant, dependent, and generally less effective problem-solving strategies than nonbattered women when asked to respond to hypothetical situations that were most likely to end in battering. Women who are less effective in solving their own problems will not only be modeling less effective problem-solving strategies, but will be unlikely to teach their children appropriate assertive, nonaggressive, problem-solving strategies.

Children exposed to family violence may have experienced psychological changes as a result of living in a violent family. Some investigators have noted the importance of examining social problem-solving abilities and interpersonal sensitivity in order to understand how violent patterns are learned (Rosenberg, 1984) and perpetuated (Emery, Kraft, Joyce, & Shaw, 1986). Rosenberg (1984) found that children with high exposure to family violence were less sensitive interpersonally than children with low exposure. This was qualified by a sex difference, with girls scoring higher in interpersonal sensitivity than boys regardless of their level of exposure to violence. Atkeson, Forehand, and Rickard (1982) have reported research showing that the extent of children's behavior problems was directly related to the amount of environmental change experienced by the children. As the amount of change increased, children perceived themselves and their parents as being less able to control their world.

The association between psychological and behavioral effects of exposure to family violence is further illustrated by an experimental study of the behavioral effects of exposure to adult verbal aggression. Repeated exposure to verbal conflict led to increased levels of both physical aggression and distress (Cummings, Iannotti, & Zahn-Waxler, 1985). Because no modeling of physical aggression occurred, the researchers suggested that the aggressive behaviors exhibited by the children may have been mediated by emotional reactivity rather than behavioral modeling. Similarly, exposure to prolonged violence between parents may influence children's affective development, which in turn, contributes to their behavior problems.

Support for these hypotheses comes from clinical observations in the Earlscourt Reception Classroom, which indicate that children from violent homes exhibit deficits in thinking through social problems and in generating appropriate solutions to social conflict situations. The teacher and child-care worker have also reported that children in the Reception Classroom often misinterpret feelings. For example, they may assume that a person making a request is angry even though the tone of voice and facial expression are calm and nonthreatening.

Academically, the children have difficulties concentrating and attending to their school work. Their apparent scattered thinking may be a result of their having learned *not* to attend when potentially anxious. An external control orientation is another noted characteristic of these children. Whereas they overestimate their own responsibility for their parents' conflict, they often underestimate their own abilities to control situations in their everyday lives.

Characteristics of Violent Families

There are a number of characteristics of violent homes that may jeopardize children's well-being and development. The dysfunctional characteristics may include lack of stability and consistency, poor problem-solving skills of the parents, salient models of aggressive responding to social problems, and the apparent success or approval of aggression as a means of conflict resolution. These aspects of family functioning, although discussed clinically, have received very little research attention as they relate to behavioral adjustment problems in children.

In violent families, it may be the ongoing unremitting conflict between the parents that poses the greatest threat to healthy adjustment in children. Rutter (1971) reported that family discord associated with separation and divorce was more critical to the development of antisocial behavior than the actual occurrence of separation and divorce. The longer the duration of marital discord, the greater the risk for the child.

Wolfe, Jaffe, Wilson, and Zak (1985) concluded that children's disturbances in social and behavioral development may be partially a function of family discord and disadvantage. Those children manifesting the most severe adjustment difficulties (as measured by the Child Behavior Checklist; Achenbach & Edelbrock, 1983) had been exposed to higher frequencies and intensities of violence. Moreover, their mothers reported more negative life events during the previous 12 months than did mothers of better adjusted children. The mothers' emotional health was also significantly related to the extent of children's behavior problems. The authors concluded that the effects on children of witnessing parental violence may be partly mediated by the mother's concurrent impairment. Hammen et al. (1987) have also reported data consistent with the notion that maternal depression can contribute in complex ways to children's dysfunctions.

Children exposed to family violence are at risk for behavioral and social–emotional adjustment problems due to their family circumstances. There is, therefore, a need for early intervention and prevention programs that address both current and potential future adjustment problems (Jaffe, Wilson & Wolfe, 1986).

A FRAMEWORK FOR FURTHER RESEARCH

There seems to be no dispute that child witnesses to family violence—at least those in shelters for battered women—are at risk of adjustment problems. However, not all forms of domestic violence are the same, and even when they do appear similar, they do not always have the same kind of impact. Some children appear to be more damaged than others by the same kind of adversity. The mechanisms that mediate the effects of family violence on child witnesses are not well understood. We hope to determine some of the ways in which the child's psychological makeup, as well as certain family factors affect the nature of the impact.

Social learning theory is frequently mentioned as a probable mechanism whereby domestic violence is perpetuated by predisposing children to regard violence as an appropriate response to social disagreements. The idea that violence is learned behavior has become almost a truism in the family violence literature (Carlson, 1984). As a result of exposure to violence between parents, children may *learn* to be assailants or victims. They may come to see violence as an appropriate form of conflict resolution, because violence has been part of the family dynamic on a regular basis. On the face of it, there is some appeal in the notion that aggressiveness in boys may be partly a consequence of having frequently observed violence during family interactions. Also, battered women often endure a violent relationship for considerable time before breaking away (Jaffe & Burris, 1982). Girls thus have ample opportunity to infer that abuse can and should be tolerated.

Although frequent exposure to family violence may encourage violence as a favored means of conflict resolution, it is becoming clear that mere exposure to violence does not inexorably produce the same consequences. A violent home situation puts children at risk, but risk factors are not absolutes that are independent of other family factors and of various psychological characteristics of the child (Rutter, 1987). Males for example, may be more susceptible to psychosocial stress from the outset (Eme, 1979). In their recent review of the empirical studies addressing direct child abuse, Kaufman and Zigler (1987) concluded that the cycle of abuse notion had been greatly exaggerated. They postulated a number of mediating factors that could affect the intergenerational transmission of violence. Some of these factors, outlined below, pertained to the child's psychological makeup.

Psychological Factors

According to Kaufman and Zigler (1987), parents who did *not* repeat the cycle of violence had clearer and more detailed memories of their own abuse. This suggests that the interpretation of the abuse at the time may influence the subsequent effects of that abuse. Rutter (1987) and Garmezy (1983) have also emphasized the importance of the individual's appraisal and cognitive processing of the stressing experience. Some children may be able to distance themselves emotionally from a bad situation. By doing so, they reduce the exposure to risk. Some children are less prone than others to internalize family strife, and are less likely to attribute causality to some deficiency in themselves. Rutter (1987) has emphasized the importance of children's concepts and feelings about themselves, about their social environment, and about their own ability to deal with challenge. To quote Rutter (1987), "It is protective to have a well established feeling of one's own worth as a person together with a confidence and conviction that one can cope successfully with life's challenges" (p.327).

Currently, there is insufficient evidence to permit the construction of a detailed protective psychological profile for children from violent families, but a positive self-concept and perceived self-efficacy in dealing with social problems would seem to be probable ingredients. The Perry Self-Efficacy Scale (Perry, Perry, & Rasmussen, 1986) taps four dimensions of perceived self-efficacy: aggression, inhibition of aggression, verbal persuasion skills, and prosocial behavior. Children are queried about their self-perceptions of efficacy in conflict and nonconflict situations. Children in our sample did not differ from normal children in nonconflict contexts, but were markedly *less* likely to view themselves as efficacious in using either aggression *or* verbal persuasion in conflict situations.

Frequent exposure to violent interparental interchanges may inhibit or interfere with the development of a variety of social skills. The most consistent correlates of social adjustment in children have been found to be: (a) alternative thinking (generating multiple potential solutions for a given problem), (b) consequential thinking (the ability to foresee potential consequences of one's actions, and to consider these in decision making), and (c) means–end thinking, (the ability to work in a goal-directed fashion) (Urbain & Kendall, 1980). The degree to which children from violent families exhibit deficits in any of these aspects of social cognition becomes an important initial question in the development of intervention programs in classes and shelters for children of battered women.

Although it is well-documented that family violence begets subsequent violence, the actual means by which aggressive dispositions are acquired is not clear. Only recently has sustained research effort been directed at the development of comprehensive theoretical models, which attempt to spell out the links between cognitive and behavioral changes by using an information processing approach. Behavioral manifestations of disorders may be caused by faulty processing at any one or all of a variety of stages of information processing. Appropriate interventions would then require an assessment of which of these stages is problematic.

McFall (1982) and Dodge (1986) have provided models of interpersonal competence and social skills in which individual characteristics interact with external influences to produce an interpretation of the social situation. This interpretation is also accompanied by responses for dealing with the dynamic that may be either adaptive or maladaptive. This model views social information processing as occurring in a number of stages. Individuals processing social situational information must be able to receive accurately and interpret the incoming stimulus information for that situation. Inappropriate responses may be due to deficits in the perception or interpretation of social situations. The next phase of the information-processing sequence involves decision skills. Individuals must generate possible responses to the situations and then decide on an appropriate response. Once a response has been chosen, the behavior must be executed and its effects on the interpersonal situation monitored. At this stage, both social behavior and self-monitoring skills are critical so that an individual can adapt behaviors to further environmental responses.

In violent families in which verbal or physical violence has been modeled as the appropriate response to social problems or interpersonal conflicts, children may be experiencing deficits at any of the stages outlined here. Children may be interpreting situations as hostile when they are not, may be unaware that nonviolent alternatives are available to them or may have difficulties in monitoring and evaluating the effectiveness of their chosen responses. In addition to deficits at any of these stages, children may be inhibited in their interactions by affective responses, deficits in social perspective-taking skills or logical thinking that could result in inappropriate behaviors and symptoms of behavioral disturbance. We are studying children's responses to hypothetical social predicaments in an attempt to tease apart the various steps in effective social problem solving. We are using a testing procedure known as the Social Information Problem Solving Interview (SIPSI) developed by Bream, Hymel, and Rubin (1986). The instrument contains descriptions of some situations that shelter children have identified as potentially challenging. The situations involve disagreements between parents, siblings, and friends. Children are asked whether a particular situation would be a problem, how they would feel, whether the disagreement was anyone's fault, and how they thought they might respond to or resolve the disagreement. Responses are coded according to the child's expectations for positive or negative social outcomes; affective reactions; attribution of blame; and types and number of problem-solving solutions. Analyses conducted to date are incomplete, but preliminary data show that the shelter children are more likely than normals to respond with "I don't know" when asked to predict their own or peers' behaviors in potential conflict situations. Taken together, the data from the Perry and SIPSI suggest that children from violent homes may be relatively inept at interpreting and coping with social conflict.

Family Factors

Kaufman and Zigler (1987) reported that the presence of a supportive relationship with one parent during childhood reduced the likelihood of a repetition of the cycle of abuse. The mechanism involved here could be practical or emotional. That is, the parent may take steps to ensure that the child is out of harm's way when violence is most likely to erupt. Alternatively, the security of a good relationship may improve the child's self-esteem and thereby protect the child through psychological adaptivity.

Maternal adjustment is thus an obvious factor that may mediate the child's adjustment. Battered women often report numerous somatic complaints, high anxiety levels, and various symptoms of depression. They are at risk for developing mental health problems, which in turn may impact on their children (Wolfe, Jaffe, Wilson & Zak, 1985). Although the immediate ill-effects of family violence are traumatic, in the long run they may be less significant than the changes and stresses in the social environment brought about by the violence. Thus, it is important to assess the relative physical and psychological stability of the mother as a potential protective factor relating to child adjustment. In our current study, we have been using the General Health Questionnaire (GHQ; Goldberg & Hillier, 1979) to assess various aspects of the mother's health, including somatic complaints and depressive symptoms. This group of mothers had a mean score of 13.3 on the GHQ. A score of 10 or more indicates high risk for physical and/or psychological health problems. Of these mothers, 73% showed significant disturbances that are not likely to improve without treatment. When maternal health is poor, mothers are likely to have less energy and fewer resources to devote to parenting. Children's behavioral, cognitive, and social adjustment may consequently suffer.

We hope to tap other sorts of potential familial mediating factors with the Home Environment Questionnaire (HEQ; Sines, Clarke, & Lauer, 1984) that assesses various aspects of the child's home, neighborhood, and school environments. The instrument is sensitive to the child's environment as opposed to the child's behaviors. For example, one of the scales measures the amount of aggression and rejection directed toward the child from within the family. Other scales on the HEQ assess Supervision—the extent to which the child's activities are monitored and structured; Affiliation—an index of parental warmth and lack of conflict within the home; and Achievement—the provision of models, supports, and encouragement of achievement within the family.

The HEQ yields scores for the subscales that can be compared with norms, where the mean is 50. Scores above 60 or below 40 are considered significant deviations. Families tested to date were, on average, low on Achievement ($M = 38.2$), and Affiliation ($M = 26.1$), high on Aggression in the home ($M = 60.0$), high on Change ($M = 70.2$), and high on Separation ($M = 61.1$)—a measure of loss of physical or emotional contact with parents or peers. Some of these homes are thus low in some features that might otherwise be protective (achievement, affiliation) and high in others that increase the risk of adjustment difficulties (aggression, change, and separation).

Ultimately, we hope to be able to determine how the social dynamics that characterize the family are reflected in children's beliefs and behaviors about how to solve social problems *outside* the family. Do witnesses to family violence show deficits as severe as those who are also victims of violence? Some children are neither recipients of, nor witnesses to violence that is nevertheless chronic in the home. In what ways do they differ from the former groups, and how, if at all, are children protected by various combinations of the family and psychological factors referred to here? Do children from the most violent backgrounds have the most impaired social skills? If so, do those with a more positive self-concept show reduced deficits?

Another mitigating variable that has been identified in the literature pertains to the availability of external support systems that encourage and reinforce a child's coping efforts (Rutter, 1983). One of the scales on the HEQ provides an index of family involvement within the community. We also hope to determine whether academic success acts as a protective experience. Rutter (1987) has suggested that task accomplishment—*broadly* defined, can improve self-esteem and self-ef-ficacy. These accomplishments can be, but need not be, academic in nature. The opportunity to succeed at *something* may be a valuable resource. Exactly why task accomplishment is protective is not well understood. It may be that children actually learn coping skills that have enduring benefits. But perhaps the particular skills are irrelevant. It may be that coping successfully and succeeding at some-thing improves self-esteem and feelings of self-efficacy. Constructs like self-es-teem need not be considered fixed properties of the individual. Children may *learn* to have feelings of hopelessness that are context specific. If so, they can also learn that some actions are effective in changing one's plight.

What Constitutes the Appropriate Control Group?

One of the major problems in interpreting previous research on family violence pertains to the difficulty of distinguishing between general predictors of child psychopathology, and those that are specifically associated with domestic violence. For example, it may be the psychological tension and inadequate parenting, rather than the presence of physical violence that create adjustment difficulties. Thus, child witnesses to family violence may not differ much, in terms of their vul-nerability, from children whose parents have been feuding or battling (nonviolent-ly) in the course of becoming separated or divorced. Hershorn and Rosenbaum (1985), for example, found that children from nonviolent but discordant families did not differ from children of battered wives on measures of conduct, nor on incidence of personality problems.

Another confounding factor relates to the fact that shelters for battered women are crisis oriented. Most of the mothers in the shelters are there for a relatively short time while they seek alternative living arrangements. The transient and stressful nature of their stay may influence their (and their children's) psychological stability. When tests are administered to shelter residents, it is not clear whether test results are attributable to the violence that resulted in their seeking the shelter, or to the stresses of residing in a shelter, or some combination of the two. For example, Wolfe, Zak, Wilson, & Jaffee (1986) found that children of former shelter residents had better social competence than current residents, in spite of the fact that former residents were more disadvantaged than current residents. It is possible that the relative stability of the former residents' living situation contributed to the improved functioning of the children in this group. Emery, Kraft, Joyce, and Shaw (1986) reported that mothers perceived their families to be more cohesive 4 months after seeking residence at a shelter than they were when help was first sought. Also, their children were viewed as having significantly fewer internalizing problems.

Yet another difficulty arises when children of sheltered mothers are compared to those from intact nonviolent families. Numerous recent studies have compared the functioning of shelter children with that of children in intact nonviolent families (Christopoulos et al., 1985; Jaffe et al., 1986a, 1986b; Wolfe et al., 1986). Hershorn and Rosenbaum (1985) included a comparison group composed of children of discordant but nonviolent couples, however there were only 12 children in this group. Wolfe, Jaffe, Wilson and Zak (1985) compared 102 children from transition houses with 96 children from nonviolent families in the community. The comparison group had significantly fewer changes in residence, and fewer marital separations than the violent group. The authors reported that violent families had fewer single parents than did the nonviolent families, however, because children from violent families were recruited from shelters for battered women, it is not clear how to interpret the designation *intact* when it is applied to families in which the mother resides in a transition house.

There is now a substantial amount of evidence that nonviolent parental conflict, including divorce, often impacts negatively on children (Long & Forehand, 1987). For this reason we believe that comparison groups like the ones in Table 6.1 are better suited to the purpose of teasing out the effects of violence from other negative family circumstances.

When physical violence becomes chronic within a family, it is highly probable that a host of other factors are also present that predispose children to adjustment difficulties. For this reason, comparing children in Group 1 (see Table 6.1) with those in Group 5 sheds little light on the role of violence in the etiology of adjustment difficulties. We believe that violence *does*, in fact, contribute significantly to children's psychological problems, as do other researchers (Emery et al., 1986), however the extent of the influence remains to be empirically documented. Rutter (1983) has speculated that the negative effects of stressful events on children may be multiplicative rather than additive. When adverse living conditions are also accompanied by frequent bouts of physical violence, the impact on children could be particularly acute. By comparing children in Groups 3, 4, and 5 with those in Groups 1 and 2, we hope to make a start toward elucidating the

TABLE 6.1
Characteristics of Target Children

	Transient	Nontransient
Violent Families	Group 1 Children of mothers in shelters for battered women	Group 2 Children of parents identified for treatment because of violence in the home
Nonviolent Families	Group 3 Children of mothers in shelters because of housing problems rather than violence	Group 4 Children from stable, single-parent (i.e., mother-only) families Group 5 Children from intact, stable families

specific influence of family violence on children's psychological adjustment. To date, no research has been conducted that utilized comparison Groups 2, 3, or 4.

To summarize, we hypothesize that some familial and psychological factors may be protective in that they reduce children's susceptibility to adjustment problems that may arise as a consequence of domestic violence. Among the variables we are specifically investigating are: (a) mothers' physical and psychological stability; (b) features of the home environment; (c) children's personality features, including self-concept, perceived self-efficacy, and affective responsivity; (d) children's social problem-solving skills; and (e) academic achievement. If the various internal and external factors mentioned above are protective, then an important question to ask is what sorts of experiences can be provided that will strengthen or encourage protective factors for children in high-risk situations.

EXISTING INTERVENTION PROGRAMS

To date, the responsibility for programming for children who experience inter-parental violence has been left to shelter workers. Because most shelters in Ontario did not receive secure funding for child-care worker positions and programs until March 1987 (via new government initiatives), services for these children have not been abundant or well developed. Nevertheless, many shelter workers perceive these children to be at risk for social and emotional problems, and have attempted to provide programs to meet their needs.

Survey of Children's Programming in Shelters

In order to assess the extent and type of children's programming in shelters, we conducted a survey of all (n = 23) shelters for battered women and their children in South Central Ontario. We were able to conduct a telephone interview with the child-care workers from 19 of these shelters. The child-care workers at the four other shelters could not be contacted for an interview during the time of the survey.

Most of these shelters have a total capacity of 20–30 residents, with a range from 11 to 86. This sample of shelters served between 148 and 536 children last year with a mean of 260 children. Some shelters have age restrictions on the children they accept, the most common being no male children over the age of 16. All but one shelter reported having at least one child-care position, most of which are full time. The shelters have had child-care workers for an average of 3 years (range 0–10 years). Until this year, the majority of child-care positions were funded by time-limited government grants. Only one quarter of the shelters reported having child-care workers available throughout the entire week. Although the majority of the shelters have some budget for the child-care programs, many report that these funds are inadequate.

All shelters with a child-care worker provide recreational opportunities such as outings and spontaneous games and crafts. Few shelters (16%), however, have a formalized weekly recreational program. In addition, the shelters with a child-care worker provide some form of therapeutic intervention with the children. Child-care interventions minimally consist of informal opportunities for the children to discuss the violence they have experienced and their move to the shelter. The most common therapeutic components are an intake interview, individual counseling with children, and children's discussion groups. Within the individual counseling and group sessions, a variety of issues relating to family violence and its effects on children are discussed. These issues (and the percentage of shelters that reported addressing them) are as follows: identifying feelings (90%), building self-esteem (84%), dealing with attitudes toward violence (84%), dealing with one's anger (79%), preventing abuse and acquiring basic safety skills (79%), changing behavior (74%), problem solving (74%), dealing with feelings of responsibility for violence (74%), coping with concerns about the family (74%), exploring sexual stereotypes (68%), and identifying and using social support (64%).

In addition to the specific programs for children, some interventions within the shelters focus on maternal adjustment and the mother–child relationship. These include the following: groups for mothers and their children (16%), family counseling with mothers and their children (32%), and parenting groups (47%). The recreational activities for mothers and their children provide an informal forum in which shelter staff can model positive interaction between adults and children while allowing the mothers to spend leisure time with their children. For example, Interval House in Toronto is conducting activity sessions with mothers and their children with a focus on family problem-solving and relational issues.

It is clear from the survey that the needs of children in shelters in South Central Ontario are now being considered and addressed with a range of recreational and therapeutic programs. Although the majority of shelters provide some programming for children, only some of the shelters have documentation on their programming (37%) and even fewer (26%) evaluate them. As the needs of children of battered women become more clearly understood through research, it will be important to develop and evaluate the effectiveness of programs that attempt to address those needs.

Examples of Programs for Children of Battered Women

Although shelters have been the primary providers of interventions with children from violent homes, there are a number of other settings in which programming can be provided. For the past 5 years the Earlscourt Child and Family Centre, in conjunction with the Toronto Board of Education, has operated a Reception Classroom for children staying in two downtown Toronto shelters. The classroom is staffed by a special education teacher and a child-care worker, with the objective of meeting both the academic and social/emotional needs of children of battered women (Pepler & Kates, 1987). In conjunction with individualized educational programming, the classroom also provides social–emotional support for the children by providing individual on-the-spot counseling, informal group discussions, social skills training, and a weekly after-school activity program.

In the London, Ontario area, a program has been developed to meet the needs of children who have witnessed interparental violence and have recently lived in shelters (Jaffe, Wilson, & Wolfe, 1986). This 10-week group counseling program focuses on the following topics: (a) identifying feelings; (b) dealing with one's own anger; (c) prevention of child abuse and acquiring basic safety skills; (d) identifying/using social supports; (e) social competence and self-concept; (f) dealing with feelings of responsibility for violence in the family; (g) coping with wishes about the family and dealing with repeated separations or uncertainty about future plans; and (h) exploring sexual stereotypes and myths about men and women. Preliminary data indicate that these group counseling sessions have resulted in positive changes in children's attitudes toward violence and perceptions of themselves (Jaffe, Wilson, & Wolfe, 1986).

Components of Programs for Children of Battered Women

It is noteworthy that many program components reflect some assumptions about the psychological consequences of family violence that are similar to the hypotheses our research is addressing. For example, many shelters have identified affect as an area of concern and have devised strategies for helping children identify emotions. The Reception Classroom staff have also identified affect as an area of concern with these children and have sought opportunities to discuss feelings and emotions in the context of regular classroom activities. The London group counseling program addresses affect in two segments—one dealing with the general identification of feelings and another dealing with anger.

Another area of concern is the potential problem-solving deficit of children from homes in which aggressive problem-solving strategies have been modeled. Some shelter staff have identified problem solving as a target issue for these children and have incorporated problem solving as a topic for discussion in both individual and group counseling sessions. The Reception Classroom staff have designed and implemented a social skills training program that systematically teaches children nonaggressive strategies for solving social problems. In the London group counseling sessions, the individual topics are approached from a mutual problem-solving perspective and one session specifically focuses on social competence.

Clinical impressions suggest that children of battered women often blame themselves for their parents' violence and consequently feel responsible for solving parental disputes. Because these children are unable to solve their parents' problems, they may feel less control over their lives in general. In response to this, shelter workers, staff in the Reception Classroom, and counselors in the London group intervention program focus on dispelling the children's belief that they are responsible for parental conflict. Additionally, they encourage the children to increase their feelings of control by taking responsibility for themselves and their own safety.

Although some shelter staff and mothers have expressed concerns regarding the children's ability to cope with school work, this has been largely overlooked in both the research and interventions with children of battered women. Shelter workers are frequently not in a position to seek appropriate remedial education for children with academic deficits. In Toronto's Huron Street School Reception Classroom, the teacher and child-care worker are able to tailor individual academic programs to meet the specific needs of individual children. To our knowledge, however, this is the only such setting in Canada.

CHALLENGES TO EFFECTIVE SERVICE

Crisis Intervention

To date, children from violent homes have had limited programming available to address their needs. Most of the services have been crisis oriented, and are available only during the child's stay in the shelter. These limited programs remain underfunded and understaffed. Further research and evaluation is required to determine both children's needs and the effectiveness of programs that are being developed to meet their needs. Programs need not be confined to shelters. School boards could provide more services to these children based on either a Reception Classroom model or on the basis of individual needs assessment within a regular school setting. In addition, family clinics and children's mental health centers could provide assessments, counseling, and advocacy for mothers and children from violent homes.

Within the shelters, more could be done in the way of programming by enhancing mother–child interactions, modeling positive parenting skills, providing individual counseling and support to both mothers and children, and by teaching family problem-solving skills. Due to the transient nature of this population, interventions aimed at psychological well-being have been provided primarily on an informal basis, both in shelters and the Reception Classroom. Counseling for children has taken place individually or in groups, in the context of recreational or daily activities. The Reception Classroom has tried to provide a more formal social skills training program, but it has been difficult to develop a standard curriculum as children remain in the classroom for varying lengths of time.

Children who are in shelters are in crisis and cannot be expected to make major behavioral or academic gains. However, such gains could be expedited if assessment services were available during the child's stay at the shelter, because the appropriate academic or behavioral services could be identified and made available once the family is no longer in crisis. Many shelters have identified this as a gap in services.

Secondary Interventions

Children who reside in shelters for battered women represent only a small proportion of the actual number of children who experience interparental violence. Therefore, services need to be developed to reach beyond the shelters to children who are known to be at risk because of interparental violence. This group may include children who have been, but are no longer residing in shelters, as well as children who are known to be living in violent homes, but whose mothers have not sought the services of a shelter. At the secondary level, shelter staff would like to be able to provide follow-up counseling and support groups for mothers and children who have left the shelters, as well as community outreach to violent families who have not been in shelters. Currently, very little funding has been made available for this type of work. Family clinics have provided support groups to a limited extent, but other social service agencies have been slow to recognize this need. School boards need to be aware of this largely unidentified population and seek to make appropriate referrals.

Secondary intervention programs could address family functioning by providing individual counseling for mothers, fathers, and children, providing opportunities for parent training, and enhancing parent–child communication and problem solving. At the same time, academic needs assessment and appropriate school placements could be provided.

Primary Prevention

Within Ontario, it has been estimated that as many as 133,000 children may be exposed to interparental violence (Kincaid, 1982). Most of these children would not be identified as belonging to an at-risk group. It is therefore essential that primary prevention programs be developed to reach these children and to help break the cycle of violence. In addition, societal attitudes toward violence are only beginning to change and more effort needs to be directed at helping children develop attitudes that do not condone violence.

One avenue for primary prevention programs would be the educational system as children spend a great deal of their time in school and school boards have a responsibility to educate children about the laws against violence in our society. In addition, schools are in a position to provide children with both role models and training for appropriate social problem solving. An example of a successful primary prevention program is that of the Lincoln County Board of Education in St. Catharines. They have developed a comprehensive Kindergarten to Grade 12 curriculum aimed at preventing child abuse, sexual assault, and family violence. Another avenue for the provision of primary prevention programs would be through the shelters because shelters workers have expertise regarding policy setting and program development. At present, however, shelter workers do not have adequate time or funds to fulfill this role.

SUMMARY

Although the past decade has evidenced an increase in both the awareness of the needs and the provision of services for children exposed to family violence, it is clear that there are still major gaps in our understanding of and our programming for this population. Although it is important to improve interventions available to children in shelters, it is also essential to reach those children that would otherwise never come to the attention of the helping professions. Ultimately, we hope that research findings will generate some guidelines for the development of programs at all levels of service delivery, and thereby reduce the problem of family violence within our society.

ACKNOWLEDGMENTS

The preparation of the chapter was supported, in part, by a grant from the Ontario Ministry of Community and Social Services. The authors are grateful to the shelters for battered women for supplying information about existing programs for children and mothers. The role of Earlscourt Child and Family Centre, Toronto, is also recognized by Michele Kates, Reet Mae and Debra Pepler who were employed there at the time of writing this chapter.

7

Helping With the Termination of an Assaultive Relationship

P. Lynn McDonald
University of Calgary

Few issues have posed more of an intellectual puzzle in the literature on domestic violence than that of terminating the assaultive relationship. The enduring issue has been typically framed as "Why do battered women remain in relationships with abusive mates?" (Aguirre, 1985; Dobash & Dobash, 1979; Ferraro & Johnson, 1983; Gelles, 1976; Giles-Sims, 1983; Langley & Levy, 1977; Martin, 1976; Pagelow, 1981; Pahl, 1985; Walker, 1979). No one has inquired as to why abused women do or do not leave their mates.

The elementary assumption behind this question is that any reasonable individual having been abused by another person would logically avoid being victimized again (Gelles, 1976). Moreover, most experts maintain that once assault has occurred within a relationship it will become more frequent and severe over time (Dobash & Dobash, 1979; Pagelow, 1981; Walker, 1984b). Even more chilling is the fact that the assaultive relationship can end in death (Browne, 1980; Chimbo, cited in MacLeod, 1979; MacLeod, 1980). Yet the extant studies indicate that anywhere from 33% to 70% of women (mainly those leaving shelters) return to their abusers (Giles-Sims, 1983; MacLeod, 1980; McDonald, Chisholm, Peressini, & Smillie, 1986; Rosenbaum & O'Leary, 1981b; Sample Survey and Data Bank Unit, 1984; Snyder & Scheer, 1981; Stone, 1984). How many women never leave an assaultive relationship is a matter of pure speculation.

Understanding why women do not leave assaultive relationships presumably sheds light on the obstacles and challenges facing women leaving such relationships and has implications for the interventions and the services required to facilitate the process. By focusing on those women who do not leave abusive relationships and by comparing them to those women who do successfully escape, social scientists are only now beginning to comprehend the complexities involved in terminating a violent relationship. In this chapter, the explanations of why women leave or stay with their abusers are reviewed in terms of what types of interventions and services are required. The major programs and services currently available are evaluated according to the women's identified needs and the chapter concludes with comments about the future research agenda.

EXPLANATIONS FOR STAYING OR LEAVING

The explanations proposed to account for why women stay or leave a violent partner are derived from the existing theories developed to explain the causes of wife abuse. The theories generally fall into two broad categories—the psychological theories and the sociological theories. Psychological approaches locate the problem within the concerned individuals and seek to explain the woman's behavior in terms of deviance or pathological behavior (Loseke & Cahill, 1984; Pahl, 1985). Explanations falling under the psychological umbrella include the masochism thesis, the presence of mental illness, personality traits including unique feminine characteristics, learning theory, and the psychological responses to victimization. The sociological approach locates the problem in a broader social structural context and focuses on the whole social situation within which the violence takes place. Explanations in this category include interactional theories of family systems, the lack of concrete resources, and the inadequate responses of informal support systems and formal health and social services.

Psychological Explanations

Masochism

The masochism thesis was borrowed from Freud's concept of moral masochism that originated in sadism that was turned around and directed at oneself (Freud, 1965). Several early researchers in domestic violence used this concept to explain why women would not leave an abusive relationship (Faulk, 1974; Shainess, 1979; Snell, Rosenwald, & Robey, 1964; Waites, 1978). Snell et al. observed that the wives of 37 men charged with assault and battering had a masochistic need that their husbands' aggression fulfilled. Waites (1977–1978) and Shainess (1979), both feminists, used the concept of masochism to explain why women did not leave their batterers but attempted to blame other sources for the masochistic behavior. Waites (1977–1978) attributed the problem of masochistic behavior to social factors and fixed ideologies about the nature of women that made masochistic behavior the logical response. Shainess (1979) laid the blame on gender restrictions in society that have played a part in the evolution of "a submissive and self-destructive style which does indeed increase their (women's) vulnerability to violence" (p. 188). Faulk (1974) asserted that the husband loses control because of his wife; he has neither the will to resist her provocation nor to accept responsibility for his behavior.

The result of these earlier psychoanalytic applications to terminating the abusive relationship was the belief that the women sought out mental or physical abuse as a life-long pattern and that they actually enjoyed the abuse. To put an end to the problem meant psychotherapy for the woman's flawed character because if she ended the relationship she would seek out another abusive situation (Waites, 1977–1978).

There is no evidence to support the infamous masochism hypothesis and a fair bit of evidence to the contrary. Caplan (1984) has put forward a compelling argument that women's apparent masochism can be equally explained by understanding healthy, human motivation. Star (1978) compared nonabused women to abused women and concluded that passivity, not masochism, was the personality trait underlying the endurance of physical abuse. In most studies, less than 7% of the women who were repeatedly battered believed they deserved the abuse (Giles-Sims, 1983; McDonald et al., 1986; Pagelow, 1981; Walker, 1984a & 1984b). There is little convincing evidence to suggest that abused women bounce from one assaultive relationship to the next. The highest figure reported in the literature for entering a second assaultive relationship is 33% (Pagelow, 1981) and the lowest is 3% (McDonald et al., 1986); a rather wide divergence that is particularly suspect because the same interview schedules were used in both studies. Most of the women in these studies reported that they did not recall any display of violence until long after relationships were established.

Feminine Attributes

Attributes commonly regarded as feminine have been postulated to be obstacles preventing the termination of assaultive relationships. For example, women who stay in abusive relationships are said to be emotionally dependent on their batterers (Dobash & Dobash, 1979; Fleming, 1979; Freeman, 1979; Langley & Levy, 1977; Moore, 1979; Pizzey, 1974; Rounsaville, 1978; Roy, 1977), to have a poor self-image or low self-esteem (Carlson, 1977; Martin, 1976; Ridington, 1977–1978a & 1977–1978b; Star, 1978; Truninger, 1971), and to hold traditional values about women's place in society (Langley & Levy, 1977; Waites, 1977–1978; Walker, 1984b).

There have been no actual tests of the correlation between staying in a relationship and women's emotional dependency on their abusers. However, the women themselves have reported that they frequently love the batterer and cherish their nonviolent times together. Many have reported the jealousy, possessiveness, and attempts at isolation on the part of their abusers as initial positives at the beginning of a relationship. They noted the desirable aspects of the sporadic periods of closeness that follow battering incidents even though these become fewer and shorter. Many men have tried to explain their abusive behavior and have made promises to quit, offering the women hope and thereby keeping them attached to the relationship (Ferraro & Johnson, 1983; Giles-Sims, 1983; MacLeod, 1987; Pagelow, 1981; Pahl, 1985; Walker, 1984b). Dutton and Painter (1981) have argued that, as the relationship continues, the women organize their entire lives around the demands of the abuser in order to avoid future violence that in turn isolates them and eliminates the development of outside supportive relationships that could assist them in eventually leaving the relationship.

Rounsaville (1978) has offered as evidence that 44% of the women in his study reported that the first abuse occurred either during the honeymoon (time of close intimacy) or at the time of the birth of the first child (decreased time of intimacy) as indications of the importance of intimacy issues in abuse. This pattern has also been found in a number of other studies (Giles-Sims, 1983; McDonald et al, 1986; Pagelow, 1981; Walker, 1984b). He also found that possessiveness and sexual jealousy were frequently found in descriptions of women's batterers (Rounsaville, 1978). Walker (1984b) discovered that 56% of the women in her study did experience the loving contrition phase after the acute battering incident that was hypothesized to provide positive reinforcement for staying in the relationship.

The findings on the self-esteem of battered women are somewhat mixed. Walker (1984b) reported that the women's perceptions of levels of self-esteem were actually high. She speculated that the abused women developed a positive sense of self from having survived a violent relationship that caused them to believe that they were equal to or better than others (Walker, 1984b). The London Battered Women's Advocacy Clinic found the opposite. The women attending this agency had lower self-esteem than a comparison group of physically handicapped adults (London Battered Women's Advocacy Clinic Inc., 1985). Although the notion that battered women have low self-esteem is well entrenched in the domestic violence literature, there have been very few actual tests of the hypothesis suggesting that conclusive research remains to be done.

Traditional ideology covering such beliefs as (a) divorce is stigma (Dobash & Dobash, 1979; Dutton & Painter, 1981; Langley & Levy, 1977; Moore, 1979; Pagelow, 1981; Walker, 1979); (b) the children need their father (Dobash & Dobash, 1979; Ferraro & Johnson, 1983); (c) the women are responsible for their mates behavior (Langley & Levy, 1977; Martin 1978); and (d) the women feel embarrassed for their family (Ball & Wyman, 1977–1978) has been hypothesized as keeping women in the assaultive relationship.

A close reading of the domestic violence literature provides limited empirical support for this perspective. Pagelow (1981), in a direct test of the hypothesis, revealed that the number of children (the more children, the more traditional the family), previous divorce, and having traditional parents only explained 17% of the variance of length of stay after the first assault. Rosenbaum and O'Leary (1981a) compared abused women (those receiving individual counseling and those receiving counseling in couples) with those women in nonviolent, discordant families and women in marriages rated as satisfactory. The women in the satisfactory marriages were the most conservative according to the Attitudes Towards

Women Scales (Rosenbaum & O'Leary, 1981a). Walker (1984b), who used the same scale, reported that the battered women in her sample viewed themselves as more liberal in their sex-role perspectives than college females. On the other hand, the Advocacy Clinic in London found, using the BEM Sex-Role Inventory, that the clients held very traditional views regarding male–female relationships and tended to see their roles within these relationships as being well-defined (London Battered Women's Advocacy Clinic Inc., 1985). Because there has been only one real test of the relationship between traditional views and length of stay in an assaultive relationship, this explanation should be regarded with some caution.

Mental Illness

Some experts have implied that abused women must be mentally ill to remain in an assaultive relationship (Gayford, 1975; Langley & Levy, 1977; Pahl, 1985; Rosewater, 1982; Rounsaville, 1978; Star, 1978). One of the first studies of 100 women in Great Britain found that 71% of the women (all seeking shelter) were taking antidepressants and approximately 50% had attempted suicide (Gayford, 1975). In a group of self-selected psychiatric patients, all of whom were abused women, 53% of the women were diagnosed as depressives, 12% as schizophrenics, and 6% as drug abusers (Rounsaville, 1978). The author does point out, however, that only 23% of the women had been treated psychiatrically prior to entering into the assaultive relationship (Rounsaville, 1978). Rosewater (1982), using the Minnesota Multiphasic Personality Inventory (MMPI), reported that the battered women had profiles similar to other emotionally disturbed women, particularly those with schizophrenia and other diagnosis that are difficult to make. After using subscales on the MMPI, she cautioned that factors that differentiated the abused women from others were likely a response to battering. The London Advocacy Clinic found, at intake, that their sample of women exhibited anger/hostility levels equivalent to those women admitted to a psychiatric clinic (London Battered Women's Advocacy Clinic Inc, 1985). Although an important finding, the women may have had just cause to be hostile.

Overall, there has been little support for the mental illness hypothesis and few studies that take account of the women's mental health status prior to the abuse. Nevertheless, the mental illness hypothesis has not exactly fallen by the wayside. Most recently, the American Psychiatric Association has pressed for the adoption in the internationally used handbook of psychiatric nomenclature, a category called the "self-defeating personality" that according to Caplan (Vis-à-Vis, 1987), constitutes a description of the traditional woman who has been the victim of physical, sexual, or emotional abuse.

Psychological Responses to Victimization

Extensive literature has developed over the last decade on the psychological consequences of victimization. Some researchers have considered affective responses such as fear and depression (Ferraro & Johnson, 1983; McDonald et al., 1986; Pahl, 1985; Walker, 1984b), cognitive responses (Ferraro & Johnson, 1983; Porter, 1983), behavioral responses (Walker, 1984b), or all three responses (Dutton & Painter, 1981).

A number of social scientists have argued that fear of physical reprisal after leaving the relationship has prevented many women from taking action (Lieberknecht, 1978; Martin, 1976; McDonald et al., 1986; Walker, 1979). This affective response is not unfounded, because most follow-up studies have clearly shown that many women continue to be abused when they seek outside help (counseling and sheltering) and even when they terminate the abusive relationship (Berk & Newton, 1985; Giles-Sims, 1983; MacLeod, 1987, McDonald et al., 1968; Sample Survey and Data Bank Unit, 1984; Smith, 1985). Although the findings vary somewhat from the different studies, the percentage of women abused after the conclusion of an assaultive relationship hovers between a remarkable 33% to 43% range.

Walker (1979, 1984b) offered the most popular explanation for the presence of depression in her convenience sample of abused women. Using the cycle of violence paradigm with three phases—tension build-up, acute battering incident, and loving contrition phases—she has outlined how learned helplessness (Seligman, 1975) contributed to inertia in leaving the relationship. Women suffering repeated abuse come to learn that they have no control over the violence and lose motivation to change their circumstances. A lower rate of positive reinforcement from the violent mate results in more passivity from the abused women and spirals down into a depressed state. The learned helplessness contributes to depression that makes it extremely difficult for women to extricate themselves from the relationship. The breaking point supposedly comes when the cost–benefit ratio changes and the rate of positive reinforcement declines following the acute battering phases (Walker, 1984b).

Despite the enormous popularity of the Walker Cycle Theory of Violence, her own research did not support the theory. Walker (1984b) found that the women in her sample were highly depressed, but the women who had terminated their relationships with the batterer were more depressed than those women still in relationships. Walker (1984b) hypothesized that the depression was the result of terminating the relationship. These results obscure the role of depression in preventing women from leaving. She also found little support for the concept of learned helplessness. Battered women, both in and out of the relationship, saw themselves as having a great deal of control over what happened to them (Walker, 1984b).

In response to some of the problems with Walker's theory, Dutton and Painter (1981) applied the phenomenon of traumatic bonding to abused women to explain the difficulties women faced in leaving a relationship. Based on their work with battered women, the authors have suggested that victimhood of battered women is an example of a social trap where immediate payoffs obscure long-term consequences. Abused women begin the marital relationship with expectations similar to other women. With the first occurrences of abuse, which are typically infrequent and followed by contrition, wives tend to view the incidents as anomalies. Repeated assaults of increasing severity and with shorter periods of contrition trigger shifts in cognition to the realization that the violence is permanent and dangerous. Unfortunately, the women have already forged strong bonds to the abuser as a result of the repetition of the cycle of abuse and contrition. As the male gains more power based on threats of violence, the women are placed in "a position of exaggerated powerlessness and consequent depression" (Dutton, 1984b, pp. 291–292). Although an attractive theory, the authors rely heavily on the work of others to support their contentions (e.g., Walker, 1979).

Ferraro and Johnson (1983) took another tack to explain why women do not leave assaultive relationships. They postulated that women rationalize the violence that inhibits a sense of outrage and efforts to escape the abuse. In their interviews with over 100 abused women, they found six different rationalizations:

1.The appeal to the salvation ethic wherein the batterer is seen as a deeply troubled individual dependent on his wife for nurturance to survive and, therefore, must be saved by the woman;
2.The wives perceived the abuse as an event beyond the control of both spouses and blamed it on external factors (e.g., loss of job) that amounted to denying there was a victimizer;
3.The denial of injury as a rationalization;
4.The denial of victimization by believing that they had some responsibility for the abuse;
5.The denial of options because the women feared they could not make it alone and could not replace the intimacy and companionship they experienced;
6.The appeal to higher loyalties such as religion, the children, or the intact family.

Only after the rationalizations are rejected through the impact of a number of catalysts (change in level of violence, change in resources, change in the relationship, despair, change in the visibility of the violence and external definitions of the relationship), did the women begin to see themselves as true victims and make attempts to change their situation (Ferraro & Johnson, 1983). Whether the women's accounts are actual rationalizations or have some basis in reality is a moot point. As an example, some women do not have any economic resources at their disposal, which sometimes makes leaving impossible (Aguirre, 1985; Gelles, 1976).

Although victimization theories are enticing because they make intuitive sense, more systematic investigations of their explanatory power is warranted before definitive conclusions can be drawn.

Social Learning Theory

Many experts propose that witnessing violence or suffering violence teaches people to solve and deal with stress through the use of physical force. Although there has been considerable emphasis placed on the batterer learning how to be violent in his family of origin, the argument has also been put forward that many women have been abused in their own families of origin and are, therefore, likely to be more accepting of abuse from their own mates (Dutton & Browning, 1983; Schechter, 1982). As Gelles (1976) has stated, "If experience with violence can provide a role model for the offender, then perhaps it can also provide a role model for the victim" (p. 662). Indeed, many studies have collected information about the family history of battered women and have reported that a substantial proportion of the women were abused in their family of origin (Gayford, 1975; McDonald et al., 1986,; Pagelow, 1981; Walker, 1984a). For example, MacLeod (1987) reported that 39% of the sheltered women in her sample stated that they had been physically abused as children, 24% were sexually abused, and 48% were reportedly emotionally abused.

The empirical investigations of this proposition have produced mixed results. A study of 80 violent and nonviolent families showed that being a victim of parental violence and the frequency of victimization made it more likely that women would remain in violent relationships (Gelles, 1976). In contrast, Pagelow's (1981) data on 350 women who were using shelters, showed that the greater the childhood victimization, the shorter the length of stay in the assaultive relationship. Among the wives in the Rosenbaum and O'Leary (1981a) study, there were no significant differences between the abused and nonabused women on the two dimensions of victimization as a child or witnessing violence. Snyder and Fruchtman (1981), in an attempt to identify differential patterns of wife abuse, found that wives with an extensive history of violence in their families of origin were most likely to seek short-term separations only and were likely to stay with their assailants at follow-up. These findings were consistent with earlier studies (Eisenberg & Micklow, 1976; Flynn, 1977; Martin, 1978). The contradictions in findings have been attributed to differences in methodology (Gelles & Cornell, 1985) and differences in patterns of abuse (Snyder & Fruchtman, 1981).

Because a substantial proportion of women in assaultive relationships appear to have been abused in their family of origin and because the results of the major studies appear to be contradictory, it would be premature to abandon this hypothesis without further investigation. If women do learn that violence is a part of marriage that has to be endured, it is understandable why they would hesitate to leave the assaultive relationship.

Sociological Explanations

The sociological theories start from the premise of the normality of wife assault. The sociologists explain that violence against women is perpetuated by society's power structure that makes men dominant over women through the creation of unequal roles for men and women. Male dominance is seen to contribute to the cultural milieu in which the physical dominance of women is acceptable (Gelles, 1985; Martin, 1976; Pahl, 1985; Roy, 1977; Schechter, 1982; Straus, 1976). The dominance is encouraged and reinforced through structures based on male supremacy (MacLeod, 1987). From this assumption, three basic explanations have been proffered to explain the obstacles encountered in terminating an assaultive relationship—interactional dynamics of family systems, the lack of social and economic resources, and the less than adequate response of the traditional health and social service system to abused women seeking help.

Family Systems Theory

The family systems approach explains violence as a product of interdependent causal processes including the preexisting behavior patterns of system members and the system processes that lead to stability or change in patterns of behavior over time (Giles-Sims, 1983). Straus (cited in Giles-Sims, 1983) has proposed that four structural characteristics in the family are associated with wife abuse: the high level of violence in society that can carry over into the family; the socialization into violence that occurs when parents use physical punishment on children and when they use physical force on each other; the cultural norms that legitimize the use of physical force; and the sexual inequality of society. Power is the common variable that underlies all of these conditions. Generally, women have less power in society and, therefore, have fewer resources to prevent violence or to leave when violence occurs.

There are numerous versions of systems theory that focus on different features of the system depending on the proclivities of the theorists. Some researchers have viewed violence as the result of an increase of stress in the system. With a violent eruption, the system returns to a homeostatic state until the stress increases again (Hoffman, 1981; Rounsaville, 1978). Others have focused on the balance of family power wherein a husband feels threatened by a more skilled wife and resorts to physical violence to maintain his dominance (Gelles, 1974; Goode, 1971; Mac-Leod, 1987; O'Brien, 1971; Steinmetz, 1977).

Giles-Sims (1983) is one of the few family systems proponents who conceptually outlined how leaving occurred. Based on her sample of sheltered women, Giles-Sims (1983) has postulated that leaving is a gradual process occurring over time, which is spurred by a choice point that is a result of new information being input into the family system. The choice point depends on the woman's recognition of the very real danger she and her children confront and recognition of her resentment toward the batterer. The boundaries of the family system expand through bridging relationships the woman develops with confidants who provide support and a link between the original family system and the larger social system. As Giles-Sims (1983) has noted, there is a conflict between the family system and the new emerging system at this juncture and the outcome depends on the strength of the goals within the two opposed systems and within the woman. Most importantly, without a new system to become involved in and without strong positive feedback to the woman, she is not likely to leave. If a woman does leave, the issue becomes whether or not she will be successful in establishing new and satisfying systems to replace the family system (Giles-Sims, 1983).

The systems perspective is just emerging although there are a number of counseling programs now in existence that exemplify the approach. New research of the systems approach is in its infancy; however, existing research has been marshalled to support its veracity. For example, leaving does appear to be a process wherein women leave numerous times prior to ending the assaultive relationship permanently, and when they finally do terminate, the major reason appears to be abject fear of the batterer and concern for the children (McDonald et al., 1986; Pagelow, 1981; Rounsaville, 1978; Sample Survey and Data Bank Unit, 1984; Walker, 1979; Women's Research Center, 1982). Gelles (1976) explicitly found that the more severe and frequent the abuse, the more likely the women would leave the relationship. Several research studies have shown that those closest to the abuse (family and friends) know about it and respond to it (Bowker, 1983; Gelles, 1974; Kuhl, 1982; Pahl, 1985; Walker, 1979), providing some support for the boundary spanning function of friends. Other studies have also shown that the women do come into conflict with their family system when they reach out to formal and informal systems (Berk, Newton, & Berk, 1986; Kuhl, 1982). Those studies that have followed up abused women who have ended their assaultive relationships detail how difficult it is to establish a new and separate family system (Giles-Sims, 1983; McDonald et al., 1986; Walker, 1984b).

The fact remains, however, that there have been few systematic studies involving data collection from all members of the family and observation over time of the entire process. Most explanations have been reconstructed from the accounts of women using shelters that may not pertain to those women who use other means to end the partnership.

The Resources of the Women

Women's economic dependence on their abusers has frequently been put forward as one of the major obstacles preventing them from leaving the relationship (Aguirre, 1985; Dobash & Dobash, 1979; Fleming, 1979; Langley & Levy, 1977; Martin, 1976, Pagelow, 1981; Ridington, 1977–1978b; Roy, 1977). Gelles (1976) has argued that the fewer resources a wife has in her marriage (education, occupational status, access to money), the fewer alternatives she has and the more she becomes trapped in the relationship. In his study, Gelles found that wives who stay were less likely to have completed high school and were more likely to be unemployed than those who leave. Pagelow's (1981) study was in agreement with these findings. Rounsaville (1978) subdivided his sample of 31 women into those who had left their partners and those who stayed. In defense of his family dynamics approach, he found that the availability of outside resources (fewer children to care for, higher social class, better jobs) did not discriminate between those who left their partners and those who did not. More recently, Aguirre (1985) discovered that the only significant predictor of staying in a relationship measured according to women's intentions was the women's source of income. The probability of sheltered women returning to the assaultive relationship increased substantially if their husbands were their sole source of income. Previous experiences with violence; the number of injuries experienced; and crucial factors such as alcoholism, sexual demands, or job problems were not significant predictors.

The challenge has been posed that family and friends are resources that could be used to assist women in ending the battering relationship (Loseke & Cahill, 1984). The retort has been that women who have been abused have been isolated by their violent partners from their families and friends and by their own shame (Langley & Levy, 1977; MacLeod, 1980; Pagelow, 1981; Pizzey, 1974). Support from family and friends has been reported to be the first resource abused women turn to but the response is believed to be minimal on the grounds that family violence is a private affair, is condoned, or because family and friends fear the violence may be directed at them (Pagelow, 1981). Pagelow questioned the women in her sample about family and friends and reported that slightly over 50% of the women received some form of help, 13% received advice, and 29% said there was no help given. The problem with the help was that it was short-lived. In a study of 420 women who sought help from domestic violence programs, 70% noted that other family members knew of the violence and about 29% were helped (Kuhl, 1982). Of the women's friends, 70% were aware as well, with approximately 40% of the women receiving some type of support (Kuhl, 1982). The Regina study indicated that 53% of the women had a good friend with whom they could discuss almost anything (Sample Survey and Data Bank Unit, 1984). A British study found that 74% of the women asked their families for help after staying in a refuge and 48% rated the contact as helpful (Pahl, 1985). In the same study, 95% asked friends and neighbors for help and 93% rated the resource as helpful.

In short, it appears that there is some empirical support for the economic dependency thesis. The lack of informal help from family and friends as a reason for not terminating an abusive relationship receives only qualified support because friends, more than family, do seem to rise to the occasion and help the abused women. Exactly how they help and how long they can help is unknown.

Formal System Responses

The traditional service system, it has been claimed, provides little, if any, assistance to battered women. Bureaucratic procedures and agency mandates to preserve family stability and the behavior of professionals (sexism) discourage battered women who attempt to leave their violent mates (Bass & Rice, 1979; Bowker & Maurer, 1987; Burris & Jaffe, 1984; Dobash & Dobash, 1979; Ford, 1983; Hendricks & Meagher, 1986; Hofeller, 1982; Martin, 1976; Pizzey, 1974; Truninger, 1971). Several social scientists underscore the emergence of the shelter movement to meet the ignored needs of abused women as evidence of the woeful performance of the traditional service system. One of the greatest fears of shelter advocates is that the traditional social service system will take over the shelters (see Chapter 8 for a discussion of this issue).

Most of the empirical evidence tends to support these allegations. Studies of physicians and other medical personnel have indicated that this group of professionals do not ask about abuse (Pagelow, 1981; Stark, Flitcraft, & Frazier, 1979) and are the least likely to identify abused women (Burris & Jaffe, 1984). Women themselves rate medical personnel as one of the least helpful groups (Bowker & Maurer, 1987; Dobash, Dobash, & Cavanaugh, 1985; Frieze, Knoble, Washburn, & Zomnir, 1980). In a very recent study of 1,000 abused women who responded to *Women's Day* magazine, medical personnel were found to be used frequently by the women but were seen as less effective than almost all the other professions (Bowker & Maurer, 1987).

Much has been written about the unwillingness of police to both attend family disputes and to take legal action on behalf of battered women (Berk & Newton, 1985; Dolon, Hendricks, & Meagher, 1986; Dutton, 1987; Levens & Dutton, 1980; Sherman & Berk, 1984a; Ursel & Farough, 1986; Women's Research Center, 1982). The ratings of the helpfulness of police vary from country to country. The ratings are reportedly high in Great Britain (Pahl, 1985) and low in the United States (Bowker & Maurer, 1987). There is mounting evidence that arrest does deter repeat wife assault (Berk & Newton, 1985; Sherman & Berk, 1984b) but whether or not this is a function of the women leaving the relationship is not known (Dutton, 1987).

Social service professionals have been used by 40% to 75% of battered women and have been rated as helpful between 50% and 75% of the time (Bowker & Maurer, 1987; Burris & Jaffe, 1984; Pahl, 1985). In a Canadian study, social workers were most likely to offer counseling, whereas psychologists tried to heighten the women's awareness of their rights and encouraged temporary separation from the assailant (Burris & Jaffe, 1984). Dobash, Dobash and Cavanaugh (1985) uncovered an interesting pattern in the responses of social workers to abused women. They noted that there were two responses made by all professionals— supportive (listening, sympathy, giving credence) and challenging (confronting the violence, helping women to escape). Women tended to ask for support at the beginning of the violence and moved toward more challenging requests as they became veterans of the abuse. The social workers tended to respond in supportive ways and were rarely challenging, which is to say they were not particularly helpful if the women wanted to end the relationship.

Lawyers have been rated as effective by 50% to 75% of the women in at least two studies, whereas the clergy have not been viewed as effective at all (Bowker

& Maurer, 1987; Pahl, 1985). Aguirre (1985), in a direct test of the effect of service use on the decision to stay or leave the abusive relationship by women in a shelter, found that none of the services utilized (legal, employment, job training, counseling, children, and housing referrals) were associated with the decision of women to leave their husbands.

Although shelters are not considered traditional, it is worth noting that they do not appear to be a main factor in terminating the assaultive relationship. Stone (1984), in a study of 133 women using a rural shelter, reported that 58% of the women chose divorce as a solution to wife abuse, but over 34% of these women had made the decision prior to going to the shelter. Only 7% made this choice while in the shelter. Aguirre (1985) reported that the women who rated the shelter as most useful were the women most likely to return to their batterers, however, the women who made the most decisions while in the shelter were more likely to terminate their relationship. In light of the rush to establish programs for abusers (MacLeod, 1987), Aguirre found that the respondents were more likely to return to their partners if the men were in counseling at the time the women left the shelter (Aguirre, 1985).

Critical Summary

Given the review of the major psychological and sociological explanations of the forces operating in the decision to stay or leave an assaultive relationship and the state of the supporting research, the overall evidence lending credence to any one perspective is less than compelling by most scientific standards (Loseke & Cahill, 1984). Taken at face value, psychological theories do not adequately explain why women leave, especially if they have become helpless, passive, traumatically bonded, or depressed. Many of the sociological theories cannot account for why women with all the resources in the world still do not leave. None of the explanations stand alone suggesting that new theoretical initiatives might be required that more closely mirror the complexities of the termination process.

Because of the difficulties attendant on accessing abused women for study, the samples tend to be small and, with few exceptions, are based on shelter populations that represent only those women seeking a specific type of help (Gelles & Cornell, 1985). When comparison groups are employed, they tend to be convenience samples of college students (Walker, 1984b) or women in therapy (Gelles, 1976; Rounsaville, 1978; Snyder & Fruchtman, 1981) and the decision to leave or stay has been approached prospectively (Aguirre, 1985) or retrospectively (Pagelow, 1981), leaving room for error. In many instances there have been few investigations of the theoretical propositions such as the cycle theory of violence, traumatic bonding, family systems theory, or service usage; however, in the urgency of meeting the needs of battered women, they have been adopted with considerable enthusiasm by the domestic violence enterprise.

The dangers of basing interventions on poorly developed theories and inadequate research are not small. The psychological explanations should be used with a certain amount of wariness because they call into question the abused woman's competency to control her own life (personality flaws, mental illness, victimhood) while the sociological explanations can be facile (change a system, provide services, change attitudes). Loseke and Cahill (1984) have argued that abused women are not particularly different from other women who are attempting to end relationships and that most of the processes they endure and the emotions they experience are quite normal. They argue that it is the experts who have developed the idea that abused women are deviant to justify the creation of a new clientele that requires very special help that only they can offer (Loseke & Cahill, 1984). Their assessment is harsh and conveniently overlooks the well-documented terror and danger abused women face in assaultive relationships and the abnormal persistence of the assailant attempting to keep the relationship intact long after separation and divorce. Nevertheless, the intent of their message should not go unheeded.

At best, the research suggests that a history of violence in the woman's family of origin, the frequency and severity of the abuse, the involvement of children in the abuse, the resources at the woman's disposal and the number of previous separations influences the woman's decision to leave the assaultive relationship. Stated another way, if a woman is to leave the relationship, she has to come to the realization that violence is not an accepted way of life and that she and her children are in genuine danger. She requires social, material and economic support to make the break. She needs to leave through a number of separations prior to the final conclusion of the relationship. Therapy that directs women to look inside of themselves for the causes of the problem would be contraindicated due to lack of support for the personality trait and mental illness approaches. Emotional support and practical help that empowers the women would appear to be more useful.

AFTER THE RELATIONSHIP ENDS

There are only a handful of studies that have followed those women who have terminated assaultive relationships (Giles-Sims, 1983; London Battered Women's Advocacy Clinic Inc., 1985; McDonald et al., 1986; Pahl, 1985; Sample Survey and Data Bank Unit, 1984). All of these studies involve women who have used shelters, with the exception of one, so there is little known about what happens to women who do not use these services and who end their assaultive relationships. Notwithstanding the paucity of studies, the results are surprisingly similar. What is abundantly clear is that to make the decision to leave is only part of the problem for assaulted women; sticking to the decision is the challenge.

The most consistent and crucial finding of all the studies is that the women were not immune to further abuse and harassment by their mates after they left the partnership. In most studies, approximately 43% of the women were subjected to continued violence, a figure that was also found in a cross-sectional investigation (Smith, 1985). Physical distance, separate residences, restraining orders, and time did not protect the women from further assaults.

Part of the abuser's persistence is undoubtedly related to the second major finding that 25% to 75% of the women still had to have contact with their ex-partners because of the fathers' access to the children (McDonald et al., 1986; Pahl, 1985; Sample Survey and Data Bank Unit, 1984). These contacts have been described as frightening and dangerous (McDonald et al., 1986; Women's Research Center, 1982).

Not surprisingly over 50% of the children in several of the studies displayed behavioral and emotional problems that added to the burdens of the women (McDonald et al., 1986; Sample Survey and Data Bank Unit, 1984). The problems were further fueled by being a one-parent family. One of the most trying experiences was finding a satisfactory income. In the British project, all of the women were on social welfare (Pahl, 1985), 85% of the women in the American study were using some type of social security (Giles-Sims, 1983), 50% of the second-stage women in a Canadian study were on welfare (McDonald et al., 1986), and 30% of the separated or divorced Regina women stated that their financial situation had worsened (Sample Survey and Data Bank Unit, 1984). A large proportion of the women felt that being on welfare was degrading and dehumanizing. About 25% of the women were working full or part time and 17% to 25% were attempting to upgrade their education. Of the women in the British study, 43% noted that loneliness was a significant problem and 63% of the second-stage women said they maintained relationships with at least one ex-resident for the purposes of mutual support (McDonald et al., 1986).

In terms of service usage, the most important services were income maintenance and social work counseling (McDonald et al., 1986; Pahl, 1985). A large proportion of the women in these studies indicated that they could not afford to go to counseling because they could not afford the transportation costs or babysitting fees.

These studies cannot be generalized but they do provide some important clues as to what women need to maintain their independence. The crisis is not over with the termination of the assaultive relationship; long-term intervention is required. First and foremost, the women need continued protection, which points to a more aggressive role for the police than currently exists because women cannot live in shelters all their lives. The latest developments in investigations of police behavior have indicated that arrest deters repeat wife assault (Berk & Newton, 1985; Dutton, 1987; Sherman & Berk, 1984a). This suggests that more arrests of men who assault their ex-wives might be in order. The justice system might reconsider the rights of fathers to visit their children in light of the rights of women and children to live in safety.

The problems of upgrading educational levels, re-entering the job market, managing children with problems, making ends meet, and fending off the batterer have driven a number of women back to their original relationships. Social service providers need to respond swiftly and with enough economic, social, and emotional resources to help the women avoid this possibility. The public requires continued prodding about the nature of wife abuse so that informal helpers are less reluctant to offer support. That many of the women have established informal mutual help relationships testifies to the importance of fostering women's networks in the community.

In Search of a Service Perspective

It is only recently that professionals have begun to realize that the time has come to move beyond the crisis of the physical violence to a focus on follow-up services for abused women and their children (Vis-à-Vis, 1987). Shelters, which have been the cornerstone for crisis intervention, have recognized this need and have instituted follow-up programs, usually delivered through group and individual counseling by professionals and/or volunteers. Some programs are only for ex-residents, whereas others include women who have never used a shelter and some programs are geared specifically toward children (Discovery House, Calgary; Transition House, St. John's). The aims of most programs are to provide emotional support and practical information, to help the women avoid further isolation, and to keep them linked to community services. A small number of shelters have come to terms with the problem of continuing violence and have established second-stage housing within existing social housing complexes that have added security to protect the women (Women in Second Stage, Winnipeg; Nellie's Second Stage House, Toronto).

Follow-up services attached to justice, social services, health, and religious programs are less in evidence. The Melfort Safe Homes follow-up program uses private safe homes in rural areas and a day center for counseling and offers follow-up support through a self-help group. The Family Services of Winnipeg runs four women's counseling groups and the Greater Montreal Social Services Centre uses a feminist group intervention program. Several hospitals have instituted health service protocols for battered women and some run out-patient groups. A few crisis units attached to police departments provide follow-up services to abused women. The London Battered Women's Advocacy Clinic runs separate groups for women who have terminated relationships. The Chicoutimi Follow-Up program helps more well-off women who have never used shelters.

Those familiar with the crisis atmosphere often observed in the delivery of direct service to abused women, know that program planning and implementation are rarely rational, orderly processes. They are frequently carried out in the absence of any hard empirical evidence as to what is effective. Programs to assist those women attempting to terminate assaultive relationships and to maintain their safety and independence from the batterer once they are free, are subject to this criticism. Programs have developed unevenly across Canada and have been appended in a piecemeal fashion to existing services (especially to shelters that not everyone uses). Programs are in very short supply, particularly in small towns and rural areas, and are probably fragmented and border on duplication. Most programs appear to operate on shoestring budgets and have to rely on volunteers to provide service (Vis-à-Vis, 1987). There have been few, if any, formal evaluations of the viability of these services. In short, there seems to be no comprehensive service perspective or calculated design in the implementation of service. The only coherent message found in the domestic violence literature and government documents is the call to communities to respond to wife abuse by providing coordinated, wide-ranging community support (MacLeod, 1987). Although a laudable plan, no one has suggested what services are essential, how they are to be coordinated, who will oversee the operation, and who will pay the bills.

Because freeing oneself from an abusive relationship is a long and arduous process, the needs of women will be wide ranging, the level of need will vary from woman to woman, and many will come for help at different points in the process. Given descriptions of the current system, it is not likely that these needs will be met in a consistent, coordinated fashion on a long-term basis.

FUTURE RESEARCH

The dangers of calling for more research is the diversion of desperately needed funds from direct service delivery. Nonetheless, effectively supporting women in their bids for independence and the maintenance of that independence in a safe and secure environment would seem to be a sensible priority. The review of the existing knowledge explaining the issues involved in the termination of an assaultive relationship are conceptually unclear, they have received very modest empirical support and, in some instances, are at risk of blaming the women for lack of action in terminating the abusive partnership. Because the majority of assaulted women ultimately consider the termination of their battering relationships, it would be important to develop comprehensive and reliable knowledge about the forces that impinge upon this decision.

An initial step would be to compare systematically the termination of assaultive relationships with the termination of nonassaultive relationships, in order to home in on the exact needs of battered women. It is possible that many of the psychological responses may be similar to those other women experience in ending relationships; for example, grief, mourning, or depression (Turner & Shapiro, 1986). The theories of victimization have been in vogue for some time, yet there is little evidence to recommend their utility. A concerted effort to unravel the victimization process would be one priority for researchers. Although systems theory is becoming the trend, the implications this approach holds for ending assaultive relationships requires immediate attention. What occurs to women following the conclusion of an assaultive relationship should be pursued further, especially in relation to their use of follow-up services and the possible ways to ensure their safety. At minimum, follow-up services should be evaluated in terms of their cost effectiveness, their organization, and their coordination.

Perhaps most importantly, there should be an intellectual overhaul of the perception that battering is a crisis that demands immediate intervention on a short-term basis. Battering is a long-term process with many crises along the way. The process does not lend itself to being carved up into prevention, intervention, and follow-up with the requisite services metered out at the appropriate junctures. This view would acknowledge the variety of needs of abused women, the different degrees of need, and would eliminate placing women into specific categories along some fictional continuum of progress that insures a false sense of failure when the women do not follow a linear path to their end goals. It might also help to solve the intellectual puzzle as to why abused women have difficulties terminating the assaultive relationship.

Transition Houses and the Problem of Family Violence

P. Lynn McDonald
University of Calgary

*T*ransition houses for battered women and their children have been argued to be an offshoot of the worldwide women's movement begun in the early 1960s (Beaudry, 1985; Schechter, 1982; Studer, 1984; Tierney, 1982). The first transition house or shelter was founded in 1971 in Great Britain and from there the practice rapidly spread throughout Europe and North America (Pizzey, 1974). Although there have been a variety of shelter models developed through this expansion, all of them have been established to meet the primary purpose of protecting women and children from immediate abuse by men. To date, there are approximately 230 first- and second-stage shelters in Canada and networks of organizations of shelters in many provinces of Canada (MacLeod, 1987). This chapter reviews the hypothesized causes of wife abuse within the context of the shelter movement and the resulting types of shelters according to their philosophies, programs, and organizational structures. Current research is considered in terms of how various models function to meet the needs of battered women and their children, and the overall impact on ending wife abuse. The chapter concludes with comments about future directions for research.

THE WOMEN'S MOVEMENT AND TRANSITION HOUSES

The rediscovery and redefinition of woman battering in the early 1970s and the social responses to this newly constructed social problem had a direct impact on the establishment of transition houses and the forms and functions they would assume today. The current interest in wife beating was not inspired by a belief that the problem had become more widespread, or because the professionals and public had become more alarmed, but because of the women's liberation movement that began in the late 1960s. The movement contributed to the identification of the existence of battered women as a social phenomenon, hitherto socially invisible. The movement, fired by a feminist ideology, significantly altered the social concept of violence against women and offered a first line of defense against abuse through the establishment of shelters outside of the traditional social service network (Ferraro, 1981; Johnson, 1981; Schechter, 1982; Studer, 1984; Tierney, 1982). As a consequence, the feminist influence has been central to, if not the cornerstone of, the shelter movement. The subsequent influx of professionals into shelters, and the unintended consequence of governmental control over them, eroded the feminist position through offering different versions of the causes of woman abuse and hence different forms of shelters. The variety of shelter models today reflect the diverse assumptions underpinning the perspectives of these two factions.

Feminist Impetus, Professional Co-optation, and Government Control

Although a number of social scientists have drawn upon diverse theories to explain how the women's movement led to the rediscovery of wife abuse, its redefinition and the concomitant solutions to the problem; there is a common thread running through their accounts: feminist influence, professional encroachment, and government co-optation (see Beaudry, 1985; Ferraro, 1981; Gelles & Straus, 1979; Johnson, 1981; Pizzey, 1974; Schechter, 1982; Shupe, Stacey, & Hazlewood, 1987; Studer, 1984; Tierney, 1982).

Ridington (1977-1978b) explained how one of the first transition houses in Canada came to open in 1973. Vancouver women, who had been involved in radical organizations representing the New Left, realized that they were oppressed and formed women's caucuses in Vancouver for consciousness raising sessions. The caucuses in turn evolved into social action projects, a health collective, and a women's information and drop-in center. Through involvement in the social action projects, the staff and volunteers were confronted with battered women requiring help that was not forthcoming from traditional social services. As a result of these developments, the Vancouver feminists offered help through the establishment of Transition House, a house like Chiswick Women's Aid founded by Pizzey as a result of similar circumstances (Ridington, 1977-1978b). Beaudry (1985) outlined a similar process that followed on the heels of the Quiet Revolution in Quebec. In Quebec, various feminist groups began to lobby on behalf of women. Women's centers were created and they too were inundated with pleas for help from battered women. The concern of the feminists led to the establishment of the first shelters in 1975 in Montreal, Sherbrooke, Port-Alfred, and Longueuil (Beaudry, 1985). This story was repeated across Canada in the 1970s.

The feminist rediscovery of wife abuse (the Americans and the British had noticed it earlier in the 1820s and again in the 1850s) uncovered the extent of the problem and made a private, supposedly individual, issue public. At the same time, the feminists posited a new version of the causes of women battering that was consistent with their ideological bent. The root of the problem could be traced to a patriarchal society wherein men abuse women in their own homes just as they do elsewhere in society in order to maintain control over them (Dobash & Dobash, 1979; Martin, 1976; Schechter, 1982). Because wife battering is an expression of a patriarchal political organization, consciousness raising and political action are required as one step in ameliorating the problem (Dobash & Dobash, 1979). Shelters organized by feminists, are therefore, viewed as short-term solutions to a much larger problem. Shelters seek to raise women's awareness about the true nature of the problem, the domination of women by men, but the end goal is to change the patriarchal structure of society. In the process of doing so, feminist shelters stress egalitarianism and informal, nonprofessional, and nonbureaucratic forms of organization.

Many professionals joined the shelter bandwagon for a variety of reasons; some out of concern (Studer, 1984), some because they now saw abuse as legitimate because services had been established (Ferraro, 1981), and others because they saw an opportunity to expand professional power (Johnson, 1981). The professionals brought a different perspective with them when they entered the shelter movement. Their perspective was closely aligned to that of conventional social services (Studer, 1984; Tierney, 1982). The traditional social service perspective focuses on the woman and her immediate situation thereby implicitly excluding the social and political structures as causes of wife abuse. Efforts are made to locate the causes of the abuse within the marital relationship itself or the dynamics of the family (see Gelles & Straus, 1979). Gondolf (1985b) has labeled this perspective the "empiricist perspective," whereas Shupe et al. (1987) called it the "family systems approach." The answers to wife abuse are quite different from consciousness raising and political action. The solutions are to render counseling or therapy to women, the abusers, or the family in the hope that tinkering with relationships will alter the family equation of abuse (Johnson, 1981, p. 831). For the professionals, shelters are an end in themselves. As would be expected, the shelters predicated on these assumptions are very similar to traditional social service agencies that are staffed by professionals, organized hierarchically, follow bureaucratic procedures, and treat the women as clients (Studer, 1984).

The final thread woven through the accounts of the shelter movement has to do with the co-optation of shelters by official control agencies that frequently represent the sexist values of the broader society (Ferraro, 1981; Johnson, 1981; Ridington, 1982; Schechter, 1982; Shupe et al., 1987; Studer, 1984; Tierney, 1982). This co-optation has been characterized as an unfortunate or unintended consequence of accepting financial support from governments and, to a lesser extent, from local service clubs. The first shelters were poorly financed and launched by crusades that often necessitated accepting funding from official agencies. The funding usually had strings attached that had direct implications for how programs would be run. Ridington (1982) explained how the process occurred in Vancouver when Transition House was co-opted by the British Columbia government in exchange for secure funding. According to Ridington (1982), the facility is no longer based in the collective feminist movement. Beaudry (1985) showed that government subsidies in Quebec were accompanied by measures to control the approaches used in the shelters. McDonald, Chisholm, Peressini, and Smillie (1986) outlined how local service clubs bought board positions allowing them to control policy decisions.

Clearly, the woman abuse problem and the solutions to the problem have been functions of the historical period in which it was recognized. The discovery and the response to wife abuse has spawned two very distinct, if not conflictual, perspectives that inform the purposes of shelters, their programs, and how they are to be organized.

Shelter Types

Currently, there are emergency transition houses, second-stage transition houses, combinations of both, specialized houses that serve native and immigrant women, and safe homes in rural areas that are available to battered women. Researchers of wife abuse have identified at least four different models for transition houses that can be used to explain most of these houses. The fourfold typology is best represented in the work of Beaudry (1985). There are two types of shelters that can be linked to the feminist perspective and two types of shelters that represent the conventional social service orientation. All models assume that the fundamental role of the shelter is to provide a safe and secure environment for the women; however the similarities end there.

The goals of the feminist type shelters split along the same lines as the groups in the feminist movement. Both groups are liberationist in purpose but vary according to radical or reformist philosophies (Studer, 1984). Radical feminism, as represented in what Beaudry (1985) called "radical liberationist" type shelters, is desirous of a total restructuring of the patriarchal society in which woman abuse is just a symptom of the condition of women as a whole. The shelter is a place in which to change, sensitize, and politicize battered women in the service of the global women's movement. The shelter is not an end in itself. The objective of this type of shelter is to involve women in the process of liberation wherein the collective aspect of the problem takes precedence over solving individual problems. Battered women are not treated as clients to be taken care of by the personnel; they are members of a collective household and are encouraged to confront the problems of women and take action. Services are at a minimum and the shelter by definition is horizontally organized, leadership is situational, and decisions are made by consensus. There are both professional and nonprofessional staff; however, the relationships are characterized by mutual sharing and learning. Government influence is avoided at all cost (Beaudry, 1985, pp. 86-107).

The reformist type shelters that Beaudry (1985) labeled "moderate liberationist" recognize that abuse is the outcome of differential power relationships between men and women that must be rectified as part of the struggle to change the social structure. The shelter is only a short-term solution in terminating abuse. The program focus is to encourage women to become independent and to solve their problems through an awareness of women's positions in society, both individually and on a group basis. Advocacy and public education are important attributes of this type of shelter. The organizational structure tends to be horizontal, such that residents have ultimate control over decisions but some coordination is necessary. The personnel is both professional and nonprofessional, and again the relationships tend to be based on mutuality. The liberationist type shelter attempts to demand services specific to wife abuse and only minimally accepts government influence (Beaudry, 1985, pp. 94-96; Studer, 1984, p. 418).

The last two types of shelters are rooted in the social service perspective (Studer, 1984) or the so-called protectionist perspective (Beaudry, 1985). These shelters diverge on the fundamental matter of women's rights. The pure protectionist shelters wish to help only women in trouble, whereas the legal protectionist shelter is prepared not only to help but also to teach women about their rights and to encourage them to use their rights.

The pure protectionist shelters generally reflect the sexist ideology of the larger society and its beliefs about the traditional role of the woman and the family. Any women experiencing difficulties including abuse can stay at the shelter. The approach is individually oriented and offers many services. These services are offered by nonprofessional staff on the basis of their own life experiences. There is a clear distinction between the women who help and the women who are helped. The organization of the shelter is hierarchical with all the power resting in the hands of the executive director and the board. Decision making is centralized and participation of the residents in the daily running of the shelter is not encouraged. This house maintains the status quo and is not adverse to government control through funding (Beaudry, 1985, pp. 89-92).

The legal protectionist houses adhere more closely to the traditional social service perspective. Women require help but they also have rights. Wife abuse is a function of failed family relationships that women no longer have to endure because of their rights. The view of wife abuse is that of the family systems approach. Relationships must be redefined and reshaped according to the tenets of scientific knowledge. Professionals and nonprofessionals staff these shelters and are committed to the delivery of a high quality of service. There is a clear distinction between the clients and counselors and the focus is on solving the problems of the individual women through individual and group counseling. Many specialized programs are available that range from child therapy programs, programs for native and other minority groups, to programs for treating the batterer. Like mainstream social services, the shelter tends to be hierarchically organized with a director who usually follows a consultative model of management. The residents often have some input into running the shelter through formal and informal groups. This type of shelter is usually fairly cooperative with the government and existing social services (Studer, 1984).

No typology, of course, is ever completely represented in the real world, and no shelter would perfectly fit into one category for long. Most shelters are in a state of flux and are likely to move back and forth across the continuum as they try to adjust to their ever changing environments and as they pursue secure funding. It would appear, however, that the social service perspective is quickly gaining ground across Canada and would appear to be the model of choice for sheltering.

Sheltering in the 1980s

According to estimates by the National Clearinghouse on Family Violence, there are approximately 208 crisis shelters in Canada, about 10 second-stage transition houses and about 12 safe-house networks available to Canadian women. MacLeod (1987), in a study of 151 shelters out of the 230 in Canada, noted that 44% of these shelters served only battered women and their children; 37% primarily cared for battered women but also admitted women with other types of problems such as drug dependency, mental health problems and housing needs; and 11% served as crisis centers accepting all women with emergencies inclusive of abuse (MacLeod, 1987, p. 50). Of MacLeod's sample, 2% offered second-stage housing providing refuge for up to 1 year, as compared to crisis transition houses that usually shelter women for only 2 to 3 weeks. Safe-house networks constitute 3% of her sample and are networks of private homes that provide short-term accommodation for battered women, usually in rural areas (MacLeod, 1987, p. 50). Although these figures indicate that all the models outlined by Beaudry (1985) are available to Canadian women, the changes in shelters as documented by MacLeod (1987) are more telling.

In her study, MacLeod (1987) indicated that there is a predominant shift toward a social service perspective in sheltering, although feminist ideals are still in evidence. For example, 67% of the houses reported that their primary goal was to provide safe shelter but 47% of the houses still included empowerment of women as a goal (MacLeod, 1987, pp. 54-55). She also noted that there has been a definite shift from collectives to a more hierarchical type of organization. Of the shelters, 84% report having a team leader or a director. Apparently, the feminist orientation is less prominent than it was in the 1970s and those remaining collectives are concentrated in Quebec with several in British Columbia and Ontario (MacLeod, 1987, p. 56). At the same time, of the 43% that made a major change in their organization, 25% indicated that they provided more professional services and another 25% had increased the number of specialized staff (MacLeod, 1987, p. 55). Not surprisingly, MacLeod noted that the whole family, including the batterer, has become the focus of attention, which is consistent with the empiricist perspective (Gondolf, 1985b) or the family systems approach (Shupe et al., 1987).

The nature of boards governing shelters has also changed. Funding for houses from provincial/territorial governments has been dependent on the shelters having a board of directors. Since the 1970s, however, the majority of these boards are no longer simply an extension of staff and their friends. Boards now represent a wide variety of high-powered professionals who function according to the principles of business. They serve as a political tool to increase visibility for the house and to garner financial support (MacLeod, 1987, p. 57).

In terms of funding, the influence of government control agencies can be seen. For example, funding based on occupancy rates, that is the per diem model, serves to restrict the services. Many shelters receive payments for room and board for women who are eligible for welfare and funding is, therefore, based on occupancy rates. Notwithstanding the implication that this is a charity model, this form of funding ignores the costs of staff salaries and maintenance, and militates against the development of services that promote education and prevention. MacLeod (1987, p. 59) found that 74% of the transition houses could not offer comprehensive services because of inadequate funds. Those government policies that demand financial support from municipalities ensure that shelters will not open in more depressed areas. Per diem allowances for Native women and their children must be collected from Indian and Northern Affairs Canada who have the final authority to approve how long the women can stay, or even if they can stay, in a shelter. Band councils, who distribute the funds to women from the reserve, request treaty numbers that violates confidentiality and the protection of the anonymity of the women (MacLeod, 1987, p. 61). In other words, the controls alluded to by the early feminists appear to have come to pass.

Having documented the rather significant trend toward a social service perspective in the delivery of shelter services, it is more than alarming that very few Canadian researchers have evaluated whether or not the diverse philosophies, programs, and structures have differing impacts on the problem. For example, the strengths of the feminist model could be argued to be that there is more commitment to the problem because of ideological zeal and a more determined effort to keep the problem in the mind of the public. The model could be seen as more supportive of mutuality that empowers women and that does not blame the victim. On the other hand, the strengths of the social service model could be argued to be stability of funding, the use of skilled persons to deal with very complex problems and stronger professional links with the community. As Canadians move closer to the social service or professional model, there is no evidence to suggest that this model is superior for delivering service. It is perhaps even more alarming that we do not have much evidence to suggest that shelters actually contribute to the termination of violence no matter what model is utilized.

WHAT THE RESEARCH SAYS

Systematic scientific inquiry has not kept pace with the growth of the shelter movement. There is very little credible research available in the public domain that specifically addresses shelters as a form of intervention. To date, researchers have primarily been interested in documenting the problem of wife abuse and its correlates or testing theories purported to explain violence (Berk, Newton, & Berk, 1986). Most existing shelter studies in Canada, the United States, and Britain have been preoccupied with demonstrating the demand for shelters to secure funding (MacLeod, 1986; Standing Committee on Health, Welfare and Social Affairs, 1982). Still, the extant literature can be classified according to three themes—those studies that focus on the needs of battered women who use shelters; those studies that consider the shelter experience in depth from inception to termination; and those studies that actually try to evaluate shelter effectiveness. At the outset, it is worth noting that most studies are single case studies; quasi-experimental designs are rare, and experimental designs are nonexistent so that results must be interpreted with caution.

The Needs of Women and Children

The only national, representative sample of transition houses is the study done by MacLeod (1987). According to her statistics, more than 42,000 women, with 55,000 children in tow, stayed in crisis shelters in 1985. Of these children, 50% were under 5 years of age. An estimated equal number of women and children were turned away because of lack of space. Although wife abuse crosses all class boundaries, the majority of the women were poor with unstable incomes, low levels of education, and were short on job experience (MacLeod, 1987, pp. 19-21). Upper and middle-class women apparently used the shelters for information, counseling, and advice, but did not stay at the shelters as readily as lower class women. Although the rural issue was not addressed in this study, 34% of the women were from out of town. Fifteen percent were Native and about 10% were immigrant women. There were no figures available for disabled women, although 29% of the existing transition houses were wheelchair accessible and 12% had staff trained in sign language. In terms of mental disability, 64% of the houses refused admittance to women with psychiatric problems, suicidal tendencies, or drug dependencies (MacLeod, 1987, pp. 21-27).

Piecing together the very few studies in Canada, which are mainly descriptive in nature, forms a picture of different groups of women apparently having different needs. Victims of abuse in rural and northern areas urgently require information and referral services (McLaughlin, 1983; Wilde-Stevens, 1985) because of lack of services and the problems of confidentiality and close friendship ties in small communities. Native women have special needs as a consequence of their different cultural views on the family, the criminal justice system, and alcoholism (LaPrairie,

1983). The discrimination they may face from other women within the shelter is not helpful (MacLeod, 1987; McDonald et al., 1986). Immigrant women are faced with language barriers, distrust of the police, fear of deportation, and discrimination from other women (MacLeod, 1987; McDonald et al., 1986; Canada, House of Commons, May 16, 1986). Those women who are physically or mentally disabled would appear to have little opportunity to use a shelter.

Of those studies that directly investigated the needs of women in terms of transition houses, the single most consistent finding was that the majority of women go to shelters for safety and security for themselves and their children (Ferraro, 1981; Ridington, 1977-1978b; Sample Survey and Data Bank Unit, 1984). This appears to be the case as well when second-stage sheltering is being considered (Barnsely, Jacobson, McIntosh, & Wintemute, 1980; Craft & Wynn, 1985; McDonald et al., 1986). Loseke and Berk (1982) in their evaluation of telephone requests to an emergency house, find that almost half of the women called for help within 1 day of an acute battering incident. At the same time, over 20% of their callers reported that the abuse had happened more than 1 week ago. This suggests that some of the women were concerned about their future. Most importantly, Loseke and Berk (1982) found that the women's needs are extremely diverse and recommend that the staff and women define the nature of the available help within the situation. In a further analysis of their data, they show that many women who call the shelter are not necessarily seeking housing at all but advice and referral information about available community services.

In assessing the needs for a second-stage shelter in New Brunswick, Craft and Wynn (1985) found that battered women rate emotional support, help in finding housing, legal advice, and protection as their most important needs. In an Alberta study of a second-stage shelter, McDonald et al. (1986) identified the most crucial need as safety, but the next most important need at time of entry was for counseling for sexually abused children. Although 88% of these women had come directly from emergency shelters, 74% believed that they had no choice about where to go short of returning to their battering environment. This same study finds that 90% of the women arrived on the shelter doorstep with only the clothes on their backs, a few toys, and a bit of money, providing evidence that even the women entering second-stage housing have not been able to meet the basic needs. Overall, the most important needs of the women in terms of the program were identified as safety, friendly environment, and 24-hour counseling to help them deal with the move and to reassure them about their children.

If the types of services offered are any indication of need, a survey of 163 American shelters found that the most frequently provided services were job counseling, women's support groups, transportation, victim education, welfare referral, and contributing to legislative reform (Colorado Association for Aid to Battered Women, 1978). MacLeod's (1987) study indicates that all houses surveyed provided help in the areas of financial assistance, health, legal assistance and housing, along with protection, referral to other services and crisis counseling. Eighty-five percent of the houses provide counseling for women and children.

Service is also offered to nonresidents. Ninety percent of the shelters provide crisis counseling to women outside of the house, 10% provide family counseling that includes the batterer, and 82% have some type of follow-up program.

A whole new shelter population has been very recently identified; namely, the children of the abused women (Roberts, 1984). MacLeod (1987) has identified 55,000 of these children. Not surprisingly, there are very few empirical studies documenting their needs. There is a growing body of literature, some of it not particularly rigorous, which suggests that witnessing the physical violence between parents is likely to affect children in the present if not the future. The range of identified effects include somatic problems, behavior problems, risk of physical abuse, and learning to model violence. These effects are usually mediated by the sex and age of the children, the intensity and frequency of the violence, and parental responses to the problem (Carlson, 1984, p. 159). The Regina study of a first-stage transition house finds that 11% of the women indicate that their children had been physically involved in the most serious incident of abuse and 21% report that their partners abused their children (Sample Survey and Data Bank Unit, 1984). The mothers also report that approximately 63% of all the children had at least one general difficulty and identified the children being withdrawn and hard to talk to as the most significant problem. Of those attending school, 49% had at least one problem while at school (Sample Survey and Data Bank Unit, 1984). A study of 630 children at an emergency shelter in Edmonton found that 87% of the children were abused or neglected (Kendall, 1985). MacLeod (1987) found that about 1,380 women who stayed in shelters in 1985 cited abuse of their children by their fathers or stepfathers as their major reason for seeking admission. That 80% of the shelters provide some counseling for resident children underscores the need.

In the Alberta study of a second-stage transition house, 80% of the women report that their children witnessed violence and 40% report that at least one of their children had been hurt (McDonald et al., 1986). The different findings may reflect the differences between those women using first- and second-stage transition houses. Approximately 72% of the second-stage women note that they had very serious concerns about their children at the time of entry to the shelter; namely, moving their children yet again and placing them in day care (McDonald et al., 1986). The state of the present research would indicate that the needs of children should be a top priority on the research agenda.

The message from the research is that a certain amount of flexibility is required on the part of shelters to meet the women's diverse set of needs. Within the Canadian context more attention must be paid to the situations of those in rural and northern areas, as well as to women with different ethnic backgrounds. Comparative studies on the needs of women seeking first-stage shelters and second-stage shelters would also appear to be necessary if shelters are going to make this distinction.

The Shelter Experience

Those studies considering the shelter experience are more in evidence; however, most of these are case studies and are therefore very difficult to summarize (Barnsley et al., 1980; Ferraro, 1981; Loseke & Berk, 1982; McDonald et al., 1986; Pagelow, 1981; Pahl, 1979; Ridington, 1977–1978a). The major issues addressed usually include the process of how women secure residency in the shelter, how they experience the programs from the perspective of their needs, their view of outside services, their relationship to other residents, and their difficulties in the shelters. As well, the studies document the experiences of the shelter staff in terms of their working environment, how they process the women, their major stresses, and their relationships to outside agencies. The data is very rich in detailing "what it is like to live or work in a shelter."

The Regina study on an emergency shelter is more than impressionistic in its findings about shelter life (Sample Survey and Data Bank Unit, 1984). This investigation finds that almost 50% of the residents did not know the shelter existed. Twenty-one percent had to wait 2 or 3 days before they could get into the house. The physical environment of the house caused some problems for the women in terms of inadequate play space for the children, crowding, and lack of privacy. However, 60% of the women felt very secure. The women appeared to be very satisfied with the staff, particularly their helpfulness, friendliness or frankness, and support. However, it is important to note that 23% of the women always or sometimes felt intimidated or defensive in their communications with staff.

Generally, the studies suggest that the majority of women using shelters appreciate and value their experiences for themselves and for their children; and that staff, although faced with incredible challenges, equally value their working experience. Most studies underscore the importance of individual counseling, the tendency of shelters to underuse community services, the problems staff have with determining eligibility criteria, the horror they witness, and the scrambling for scarce resources (Ferraro, 1981; Loseke & Berk, 1982; McDonald et al., 1986; Ridington, 1977-1978a). The studies by Ridington (1982) and Ferraro (1981) indirectly refer to the benefits of living in a feminist type shelter and the Calgary study (McDonald et al., 1986) details the repercussions of living and working in a pure protectionist type shelter. Given these mainly descriptive investigations, it is clear that more research is required to assess empirically the independent and joint contributions the various dimensions of shelter life such as specific programs, community links, organizational structure, and type of staff, make in the struggle to end violence. The time has come to evaluate empirically the components of shelter life as they have impact on the women's experiences.

Terminating Violence

Evidence indicating that shelters have a direct impact on ending violence is scant and what does exist is suspect. Different studies use different outcome measures such as whether a woman is beaten again (Giles-Sims, 1985; McDonald et al., 1986), whether she returns to the batterer (Snyder & Scheer, 1981), and sometimes both measures (Sample Survey and Data Bank, 1984). First, the two types of studies are not comparable. Second, any of those studies that use repeated violence as an outcome measure have no control groups of battered women not in shelters for comparison. Third, those studies that use living arrangements as an outcome of shelter stay do not account for the issue of physical safety when a woman returns to her mate; they do not account for a woman's change of heart to go back to her mate after being on her own for some time; and finally, if the woman is on her own, this measure does not account for the possibility of the abuser paying her a visit and beating her.

Notwithstanding these problems, there is isolated evidence to suggest shelters are contributing to the discontinuation of violence. Snyder and Scheer (1981), using data from 70 emergency shelter residents, find that at a 6-week follow-up, 55% of the women were living with their original assailants but only 12% of them were physically abused again. Giles-Sims (1985) in a study of 31 women, 4 to 6 months after residing in one shelter, found that the incidence of violence had declined as measured on the Family Conflict Tactics Scale.

In evaluating the specific goals of a second-stage program, the findings indicate that the women's fears were significantly reduced from time of entry to the time they left and at 6 month follow-up. The women had more internal control and more social independence at a 6-month follow-up compared to what they experienced when they entered the house (McDonald et al., 1986).

Bowker and Maurer (1985), with a sample of 150 newspaper selected subjects, studied evaluations by victims of strategies to end violence and concluded that shelters were important but not as significant as other strategies. The Regina study (Sample Survey and Data Bank Unit, 1984) followed up approximately 98 women at various time points after their stay in Transition House and found that approximately 28% of all 98 women were physically abused following their stay at the House. Of those women still with their partners, 31% were abused compared to 33% no longer with their partners. Aguirre (1985) reported that for a subsample of 312 respondents in the Texas Survey of Shelters, 49% of the women in the follow-up study returned to their abusive spouses. Whether these women were subsequently abused was not mentioned. In a small group of women ($N = 30$) followed up 6 months after a stay in the second stage shelter, 35% of them went on their own but almost 38% of these women eventually returned to their battering partners. Almost 50% of these women were abused again. Of those women who permanently separated, 42% were still being harassed by the batterer (McDonald et al., 1986). In perhaps the best study to date, Berk, Newton, and Berk (1986), in a two-wave panel of wife-battery victims ($N = 155$), discovered that shelters have beneficial effects in ending new violence only for battery victims who are already taking control of their lives. Otherwise, shelters may have no impact or can even trigger retaliation by the batterer for having sought shelter.

What is evident from the research about the impact on violence is that shelters probably do help. We need, however, more and better controlled studies that look at a wide variety of outcome measures. We need to test the effectiveness of different shelter models in ending violence as well as the differences between first- and second-stage shelters and the efficacy of safe homes. The effectiveness of shelters should also be tested with other intervention strategies such as counseling programs for the batterer, public education programs, and legislative changes.

CONCLUSIONS

This chapter has attempted to provide an overview of shelters as one form of intervention used to combat the problem of family violence. Feminist, professional, and governmental influences have been central factors in determining the current philosophies, programs, and administrative structures apparent in shelters today in Canada. A review of the current research suggests that there are serious gaps in our knowledge base. The needs of women and children must be more clearly delineated, particularly for those in rural and northern areas and those of varying ethnic backgrounds. Most women's experiences in shelters appear to be positive, but which experiences are more useful than others is not evident and what works for children has been poorly documented. Although there is no evidence to suggest which type of shelter is more effective, there is some empirical support that transition houses do assist in ending battering. At the same time, clear distinctions will have to be made between first and second stage shelters as to purpose and functioning if we are to best meet the needs of abused women and their children.

9

Integrating Systems: Police, Courts, and Assaulted Women

Luke J. Fusco
Wilfrid Laurier University

*E*stimates vary that between 40% and 70% of all violent crime in Canada and the United States occurs between people who live together. In Canada, these figures suggest that approximately 750,000 couples have at least one dispute involving violence each year (Dutton, 1984a). Other researchers estimate that between 10% and 50% of women living with a male partner will be assaulted during the relationship (Burris & Jaffe, 1984). Until recently, police, prosecutors, and judges, reflecting the attitudes of the public, dealt with wife beating differently from the same behavior occurring between strangers (Dobash & Dobash, 1979; Moore, 1979; Pressman, 1984; Roy, 1977). Today, police are more likely to charge batterers with a crime, but the issue remains controversial.

The assumptions upon which a question is formulated can inadvertently point the discussion in a specific direction. In the concern with and examination of wife battering, it is recognized that the need exists for assistance to all family members (including the batterer) and simultaneously that the illegal nature of the act somehow be marked. The question posed is whether a husband striking his wife is a crime or a family problem. Given this ambiguity, it follows that police, justices of the peace, prosecuting attorneys, and judges do not have clear guidelines. Should police stay out of family matters or should they lay charges? Court personnel receiving information are skeptical of the willingness (and the wisdom) of victims following through on the charges. Finally, in those instances when a case does get to court, are the judges to see the guilty husband as a criminal or as a man with marital problems? Is there, in fact, an inherent qualitative difference between violence in families and violence between strangers? Does a case involving an assaulted wife belong in family court or criminal court?

The response to these questions will determine the direction of future judicial and social policy. Most recent reports suggest that wife assault can be viewed as both a crime and as symptomatic of family problems (Burris & Jaffe, 1984). The violence itself is very much a problem for all people within the family system. To emphasize only the criminality of wife battering suggests that an adequate criminal justice response is enough. We know this is not true. But equally incomplete is a purely social service solution that all but ignores the clear violation of criminal law inherent in any and all assaultive behavior.

A review of police and court policies and an analysis of data from those programs that seek to combine law enforcement and criminal justice responses with psychological counseling and social services form the main part of this chapter. Following this, it may be possible to draw at least tentative conclusions and to see directions for future program development and research.

THE POLICE

Kennedy and Homant (1984), in their Detroit study, found that 70% of residents of shelters for battered women found the police to be helpful. Respondents in this study also saw roles for female and male officers in relation to offering understanding, preventing further violence or injury, listening, advising, calming, mediating, and arresting. Sixty percent said that they would prefer at least one policewoman coming to their assistance in the future.

Pahl (1982) found that the term *domestic dispute*, commonly used to characterize acts of physical violence toward wives, trivialized the behavior and created an attitude that saw assault as no more serious than a spat. Pahl compared this to using the word "litter" to describe all waste: from candy wrappers to toxic industrial chemicals.

The results of Pahl's research in Canterbury, England, underline the reluctance of police to become involved in a controversial offence. Those respondents who saw the police as not helpful tended to be married and living in the same house. Those women who found the police helpful were usually not married, legally separated, divorced, or living apart from their male partners. Apparently intact marriages were off-limits for police intervention. This finding held up notwithstanding the severity of injury or frequency of request for help. Finally, anecdotal responses reported by Pahl supported previously published reviews of the law that maintains women in a position of subservience and dependency (Freeman, 1980).

Ford (1983) reported on police responsiveness to requests for help from victims of wife battering in Marion County, Indiana, which includes Indianapolis. Data was obtained from a variety of sources including the police department, county sheriff's office, and the municipal courts. "Between two-thirds and three-fourths of all calls to police on conjugal fights were 'solved' by the dispatchers"

(Ford, 1983, p. 465). In other words, no police officer went to the home of the caller in the majority of cases.

Dobash and Dobash (1979) point out that police use their discretionary power to avoid making arrests or even laying charges. While recognizing the importance of police discretion in overall law enforcement, the authors noted that underenforcement in cases of violence against wives subverts justice and may even endanger lives.

Roy (1977) described a covert toleration of wife beating among police and court officials. The pattern of reluctance to intervene, fear of injury (Bowker, 1982; Police Foundation, 1977) and, in some jurisdictions, even a written policy of nonarrest in cases of domestic violence (Thorman, 1980) have combined for most of this century to exclude the official guardians of the peace from family related assaultive behavior. Berk and Loseke (1980-1981), in a California study, found that the probability of arrest actually decreased if the woman called the police for help. Bowker (1982), in a Milwaukee, Wisconsin, study found that the two most common reasons given by battered wives for contacting the police were fear for their own lives (59%) and the desire to make a statement to their husbands about ending the violence (32%).

Using factor analysis, Bowker sought to describe the characteristics that predisposed wives to call the police. A profile emerged of women who were unable to influence their husbands' behavior through their own personal strategies; women dominated by their husbands who relied mainly on passive defenses; and third, a group of women who depended on the formal help offered by police and lawyers (Bowker, 1982, pp. 483-485). Eighty-two percent of the wives asked officers to arrest their husbands but arrest occurred in only 14% of the cases.

Understandably, there was a generally low level of satisfaction with police services expressed by the battered women. A summary of this study suggests that many women who are assaulted by their husbands are unable or afraid to confront and stop the attacks on their persons. The police are seen as potentially providing physical protection and communicating directly to the violent husband that there are clear limits regarding acceptable and unacceptable, legal and illegal behavior. Bowker cited 10 other reported findings in which battered wives gave negative ratings to the police (Bowker, 1982, p. 488).

In the United States, class action suits on behalf of battered wives resulted in police departments treating domestic violence as a criminal matter in the cities of Oakland, Los Angeles, and New York and in the state of Oregon (Bowker, 1982; Morash, 1986).

The police are not the problem. Men assaulting women and society's long acceptance of this behavior surely are the problems. Directives that institute new policies can help, but police officers are part of the community and their conduct and attitude toward wife beating reflect the community's values to a great extent (Muir & LeClaire, 1984).

There is dramatic evidence of the potential benefits for and the impact of arrest on both the victims and their assailants. In the Minneapolis Domestic Violence

Experiment (Sherman & Berk, 1984b), suspects in domestic assault cases were responded to by police in one of three ways: arrested, sent from the scene for 8 hours, or given some form of advice. Suspects were assigned to each category by lottery. The study included 205 victims over an 18-month period in 1981-1982. Outcome was judged on the percentage of repeated violence over a 6-month period. Measured by either official records or victim interviews, the arrest cohort had significantly lower recidivism. The percentage of repeat violence over 6 months was 37% for the advised cohort, 33% for the sent-from-the-scene cohort, and 19% for the arrested cohort. In addition, when the victim felt that the police listened to her as well as arrested her husband, the repeat violence was reduced to 9%. The explanation of the authors is that the victims felt empowered and this empowerment had a deterrent effect on the batterer. Despite the authors' cautious interpretation of the findings, the Minneapolis Police Department changed its policy on domestic assault and required officers to submit written reports when they failed to make an arrest which was legally possible.

Jaffe, Wolfe, Telford, and Austin (1986) studied the impact of police laying charges in incidents of wife assault in London, Ontario. With virtually the same number of wife assault occurrences in the prepolicy year as during the third year of the policy, there was a 2,500% increase in the number of charges laid by police. Specifically, there were 12 arrests out of 444 occurrences in 1979 and 298 arrests out of 443 occurrences in 1983 (Jaffe, Wolfe, Telford & Austin, 1986, p. 43). Other findings showed a marked decrease in violence following arrests and much higher victim satisfaction with police response, but no significant increase in satisfaction with the Crown Attorney between 1979 and 1983. The police reaction to the change in policy was mixed. Most officers believed that a clear message was sent to the community, but a smaller minority felt that it helped reduce violence.

Muir and LeClaire (1984) studied the impact of a change in policy in favor of arrest and the initiation of assault charges at the time of the violent incident. One immediate result was a 700% increase in the number of charges laid even though the police retained their traditional discretionary power.

Follow-up of the victims of these assaults show results remarkably consistent with the attitudes and opinions expressed by the women surveyed in the Milwaukee study. The greater likelihood of charges being laid and the availability of charging as an expression of power and effectiveness was seen as both protection and deterrent (Muir & LeClaire, 1984, pp. 43-44). Of the victims, 70% expressed satisfaction with police and the prosecution of their cases (Muir & LeClaire, 1984, pp. 43-44). They were not satisfied with subsequent court action as described here.

Police officers were more dissatisfied with the change, although 40% expressed satisfaction with the new policy (10% did not respond). Reasons for police satisfaction included the expansion of discretionary power and assistance to victims. Those officers who stated that they were dissatisfied with the new policy expressed frustration with the high percentage of dropped charges. The police saw this as a waste of time when in fact the victims used their own discretion, feeling that the laying of charges was a sufficiently strong message in itself.

Many of the police officers surveyed in the Calgary study recognized a need for a different type of assistance for female victims and the general inadequacy of police alone to meet that need (Muir & LeClaire, 1984, p. 75). Levens (1978) surveyed 60 police departments in Canada and the United States and found that between 50% and 80% of time on the job is spent in social service activities. These activities included domestic calls as well as a wide range of other duties that did not involve law enforcement as the primary objective. Levens carried out a more detailed study of the Vancouver Police Department. His findings are consistent with those cited previously: no predictable response pattern to domestic calls although such calls constituted about 18% of all calls to the police and an even higher proportion of patrol officers' time because domestic calls take more time than other kinds of calls (Levens, 1978, p. 7).

The theme of frequent requests for assistance from battered wives and a generally ambivalent response from police suggests that either women who are assaulted by their husbands should stop calling the police or that the police should be trained to perceive responding quickly and effectively as legitimate and routine elements of their job.

Levens' conclusions and recommendations apply to all situations involving police and domestic violence. Specifically, Levens urged a number of actions:

1. Police must receive training that emphasizes police safety, availability, dispute management and crisis intervention, referral assessment, and links with the social service network. Implicit in this is the need for social agencies to view the police as partners who deserve respect, cooperation, information and feedback.

2. Training of police telephone operators and dispatchers to screen calls accurately to identify which require immediate police involvement, immediate social service involvement, both, or a referral to an appropriate agency.

3. Even immediate police intervention, mediation, and referral will not be sufficient in many instances. Mental health professionals including social service personnel must be available, on call, or able to accompany police to the call in the first instance (Levens, 1978, pp. 32-34).

One advantage of expanded social agency time is to take some pressure off the police. As police see family complaints routinely as assaults and more often lay charges, they should be able to turn to the social service network and the mental health system to help the family with both the short-term effects of the crisis and with long-term planning. Protection, legal advice, counseling, and therapy may all be required by various family members. Material services such as money, housing and food may be needed. An arrest, although essential, may well be but a first step.

Police–Social Service/Mental Health Teams

There is additional evidence to examine from jurisdictions where police and helping professionals have attempted to work together to provide a comprehensive range of services to victims of wife assault and their families.

Police training can include understanding of and appropriate responses to wife battering. Excellent programs, manuals, visual aids, and other resources are readily available. Reports indicate that many police forces now include related material in both recruit training and in on-going in-service courses for experienced police officers (Loving, 1981).

Experience suggests that the negative stereotypes with which police and social workers initially confront each other tend to change over time. Working toward shared goals seems to ease the natural tensions noted by a number of observers (Parkinson, 1980; Treger, 1975; 1981).

Holmes (1982), in describing a police–social work model introduced in Detroit in 1976, also referred to Parkinson's (1980) findings on sex-role stereotyping as an area of difficulty for police in dealing with domestic violence and as an area of potential conflict between police and social workers. However, in Detroit, following a 1-year pilot project, a program was instituted where a social agency (The Family Trouble Clinic) provided services to families in its offices between 8 a.m. and 5 p.m. weekdays. Between 5 p.m. and 8 a.m. on weekends, another group of family workers were on-call and went to the scene of the incident and provided office appointments or counseling over the phone as required. Holmes noted that although the team approach was seen as successful, the police must be able to make appropriate referrals. The police responded to calls initially and used their discretion in calling in the family workers. Clearly, under those circumstances police must be trained and practiced in assessing a family crisis and summmoning assistance. Holmes found that repeat calls went directly to the social agency worker rather than to the police. Families called the clinic when they recognized a crisis building and avoided a repetition of violence (Holmes, 1982, p. 225). A reduction in future violence would be sufficient reason to provide a crisis service.

In Restigouche County, New Brunswick, trained volunteers are used to assist police on a 24 hour on-call basis (Lerette, 1984). A police officer calls the volunteer to the scene of an incident; the officer observes the interaction with the family for signs of further violence and then leaves when the parties are sufficiently calm. In the typical occurrence, the officer leaves after a few minutes and calls back periodically to monitor the intervention (Lerette, 1984, p. 19). Volunteers are trained in crisis intervention and dispute resolution. If long-term services are required, the volunteers make referrals to appropriate agencies.

Calgary has a 24-hour Police Crisis Unit also utilizing volunteers who provide expert assistance in assessment and intervention in crisis situations (Police Family Crisis Intervention, 1983, pp. 46-49). Again, the crisis workers do not provide on-going family assistance but do make referrals to family agencies when such help is needed. Similiar programs also exist in Toronto, Kenora, and Regina (Police

Family Crisis Intervention, 1983). Chatham, Ontario, and Vancouver have crisis response teams that are linked with the police (Kent County Task Force on Family Violence, Chatham, Personal Communication, 1987; Ministry of Human Resources, Vancouver, B.C., Personal Communication, 1987).

The Family Consultant Service in London, Ontario, has existed for over 13 years and has been part of that city's police service since 1976 (Broemling, 1986). It is the model for comparable services in North America and abroad. Often publicized, studied, and evaluated, the Family Consultant Service has delivered crisis services on an almost round-the-clock basis every day for well over a decade. The model of police responding to the call first and then asking for the intervention of the family consultant on duty has worked quietly and effectively and proven itself as an invaluable part of human service delivery. Most cases involve family disputes although the service has expanded to include other personal problems such as psychiatric illness and suicide (Jaffe, Finlay, & Wolfe, 1984).

As suggested earlier in this chapter, the availability of family service workers does not preclude the advisability of police training in crisis management. In London, the police officers may use their own skills and knowledge of social agency resources successfully. According to Jaffe and his colleagues (1984, p. 65), only 25% of all crisis calls that could be referred to the Family Consultant Service are referred. The intervention is crisis management, problem solving and, usually, a referral for long-term work to an appropriate community resource.

Indications of success include positive attitude survey results from the police and other mental health and social service agencies in the community. Perhaps the most encouraging fact is that there has been a consistent decrease in the number of repeat calls by families to the police force. Repeat calls usually mean increased violence so "this finding underlines the importance of preventing repeat calls" (Jaffe et al., 1984, p. 66).

Jaffe et al. (1984) also reported the results of a study to determine the long-term impact of the family crisis unit on family conflicts. Although the results must be qualified (as the authors point out) because of small sample size and other methodological limitations, the findings suggest that the benefits gained in the 48 hours following the crisis incident and evident again at 3 months remain even after 3 years.

A model used in Hamilton, Ontario, in which a crisis counselor received referrals from the police but was not on immediate call also seems to have produced positive results (Knowles & Middleton, 1980). A reduction in violence, with 64% of the women surveyed saying the violence had stopped, was a strong indicator of success. It is also interesting to note that "called the police" was seen as "the most important step (taken) in dealing with the problem" (Knowles & Middleton, 1980, p. 13).

PROSECUTORS AND THE COURTS

Custom and the law long supported violence against women (Freeman, 1980; Taub, 1983). Some legal experts to this day would argue for decriminalization of domestic violence as a way to bring treatment and change to the family (Maidment, 1980). Others go further and analyze wife abuse in systems terms with an outright rejection of the offender–victim dichotomy and criminal court involvement (Benjamin & Adler, 1980).

In a fascinating and highly instructive article, Ellis presented a long and probing dialogue between herself and an imaginary prosecutor about the logic, procedures, thinking, and philosophy underlying decisions to prosecute or not to prosecute men who assault their wives (Ellis, 1984).

In a civil matter, the issue is between two individuals and the justice system provides a forum and rules with which the matter at hand can be resolved. The initiation of proceedings is up to private individuals. In criminal cases, prosecutors act for the state and bring charges on behalf of the community. A statement is made that we as a people condemn the criminal behavior and charge the offender with a crime against the community as a whole. Not only is it unnecessary for the victim to initiate the action, but charges can be laid in spite of the victim's objections if the violation of community standards is sufficiently serious. These judgments are made by justices of the peace and prosecutors.

Since July 1982, when the Canadian Parliament passed a unanimous motion recommending that police lay criminal charges in wife assault cases, most jurisdictions have moved to implement policies consistent with that motion. In the studies cited earlier, findings demonstrated that although battered wives were satisfied with police involvement, they were not so pleased with the handling of their cases in court.

It is imperative that Attorney Generals and their representatives in prosecutors' offices follow through on police information with formal charges and court appearances. Ursel and Farough (1986) demonstrate the effectiveness of such an approach in Winnipeg after a directive from the Attorney General of Manitoba to arrest and lay charges "where there were reasonable and probable grounds that an assault had taken place."

Dutton (1984a) reviewed the uncertainty and confusion with which prosecutors and justices of the peace receive, process, and act upon information about assaulted wives. Those cases that do go to court and where guilt is established usually result in lenient sentences (Dutton, 1984a, p. 59). Judge Thompson, the Senior Family Court Judge in Ontario at the time, described the conflicts created for a sentencing judge. Emphasis on the violent act as a crime might hasten the break-up of a family, while concentrating on counseling appears to minimize criminal assault. Again, the question emerges should the criminal nature of the action be the predominate consideration or should the reconciliation of the spouses (where possible) take precedence (Dutton, 1984a, pp. 56-57)?

If a policy of arresting assaultive husbands is to be established and maintained, then all other decisions that affect the spouses must be consistent. Arrest is empowerment of the woman victim. It is an act of taking her side and expressing the feelings of the community about the violence. Not to prosecute, to dismiss the matter in court, or to treat it lightly is to diminish the effect of arrest.

There is a need to coordinate the subsystems within the criminal justice system as a whole. There is also a need to integrate the criminal justice system and the mental health and social service networks. The implementation of one system does not preclude the involvement of the others. Criminal charges do not prevent people from working on their problems, including marital problems.

There is clear evidence that battered wives, their assaultive husbands, and the community at large support police and court involvement in violent domestic acts (Bowker, 1982; Jaffe, Wolfe, Telford, & Austin, 1986; Kennedy & Homant, 1984; Muir & LeClaire; 1984). Also evident is the effectiveness of immediate crisis intervention services by trained family specialists. Reduced family violence and decreased calls to police are two of the most important benefits of such programs.

The question is no longer will a program like the one in operation for 14 years in London work, but why have more communities not established similar programs?

CONCLUSIONS

Some conclusions are justified by this review of the literature:

1. Many women who are assaulted by their male domestic partners need law enforcement, power to arrest, and the usual sympathy accorded to victims by the patrol officers who arrive on the scene.
2. Police should be trained to view domestic assaults as appropriate and routine situations for police intervention. Specialized training involving the nature of domestic assault, crisis intervention, and conflict mediation would make police intervention more effective.
3. Police alone cannot meet all the needs presented in many incidents of violence toward wives. Part of the police reluctance to act in the past was based on inadequacy of response skills and lack of immediate resources.
4. Social services, including material assistance, protection, and counseling must be linked closely to the police on a daily 24-hour basis. Next day referrals to agencies that require the victim to make the initial contact are a poor substitute for an immediate response to a violent crisis.

Two critical factors underlie the historic acceptance of wife battering. One is the socialization of sex-role stereotypes. The other is a male dominant social structure in which coercion and force are legitimate control mechanisms. Some recent programs that counsel batterers seek to change these two fundamental aspects of domestic violence rather than providing quick fix solutions directed at anger or temper control (Adams, 1988; Gondolf & Russell, 1986).

In a recent Canadian study of wife abuse, Linda MacLeod (1987) defined abuse in broad terms that included psychological and emotional abuse. Gondolf and Russell warn that these nonphysical forms of abuse often will not be eliminated and may, in fact, be reinforced in treatment programs employing a narrow approach concentrating on anger control. They advocate an effort much broader than anger control, patterned after the successful treatment of alcoholics.

> Batterers, like recovered alcoholics, need long-term reeducation and monitoring. That is, "getting better" for the batterer means a lifelong committment to abstinence from abuse with many external supports. Program, community and societal efforts to curb such problems as alcohol abuse appear to be having a positive effect and this same sort of movement needs to be mounted against wife abuse. (Gondolf & Russell, 1986, p. 5)

Practitioners in the clinical area may seek a simple model of behavior control that, although controlling physical violence, ignores the critical fundamental issues of sex-role stereotyping and the sometimes abusive tactics of men attempting to control women. The growing recognition of this trap must be accompanied by a parallel movement within the larger arenas of policy formation and program development in the criminal justice system and in the social service and mental health systems. Successful treatment of batterers requires community support for broad changes in attitudes, assumptions, socialization to gender identity, and behaviors. Those who even indirectly support battering must also change. Enlightened public policy must address the view that wife assault is a crime as well as a social problem. To argue that it is only one of these is to create a false dichotomy that will prevent an adequate public response. The following policies are required in order to implement an effective dual approach to wife battering:

1. Clear guidelines must be offered to police on the importance of arresting men who assault wives.
2. Mandatory police training in the nature of wife battering and in domestic assault responses should be instituted.
3. Associations of helping professionals or interagency networks must be linked directly with police on domestic violence calls. An alternative is that social service counselors could work directly for or with the police and even be based physically in the police stations.
4. Assault charges must proceed to adjudication in criminal court. The Criminal Code does not exclude wife assault.
5. Courts may look at other aspects of the offenders situation during the sentencing process as happens in all criminal cases.
6. As therapeutic interventions are refined, tested, and proven successful, and as other forms of protection are developed (Pressman, 1984; Sinclair, 1985),

their availability should not be used to justify a de-emphasis on the totally unacceptable and criminal nature of assault on women.

7. All public responses to wife assault should be consistent with the two messages that it is a crime requiring legal action and a family problem sometimes requiring social or psychological intervention.

FUTURE RESEARCH

The studies cited in this chapter strongly suggest that police and judicial responses that support the victim and arrest and prosecute the batterer are viewed positively by most women and some men. These criminal justice reactions may also reduce future incidents of violence.

Quantitative studies comparing indices of wife assault prior to and following dramatic changes in police, prosecutorial, and judicial practices and the availability of immediate crisis intervention around the clock must be carried out in order to evaluate the effects of the policy changes.

Qualitative research also should be done with battered wives. Descriptions by these women of their experiences before and after formal legal and counseling interventions would be instructive. Consistent with the idea that change beyond behavior control is necessary before the pattern of wife abuse is stopped is the need to study the changing quality of power sharing between husbands and wives or even men and women in other contexts.

Any less ambitious goals do not address the basic problem of wife assault.

10

What We Know About Preventing Wife Assault

Anne Westhues
Wilfrid Laurier University

*A*lthough wife assault is a problem that has long been with us, it is only recently that it has been accepted as a social, or public problem rather than an individual, or private one. One consequence of this is that funding has become available for research, and we now have some understanding of the prevalence, etiology, and treatment of wife assault. Although the nature of the problem prevents the data from being definitive, research suggests that in Canada 1 woman in 10 (MacLeod, 1980) and in the United States 1 woman in 6 (Straus, Gelles, & Steinmetz, 1980) has been physically or sexually abused by her partner. When this definition of battering is broadened to include verbal abuse, a recent report (MacLeod, 1987) suggests that the prevalence in Canada increases to 1 woman in 8.

Another part of the response to the growing evidence of the magnitude and severity of wife assault has been to build a network of places of safety that would give the victims of abuse—women and children—protection from being battered. In Canada, for example, no shelters existed for women before 1972. By now, there are 275 agencies offering accommodation and services in a variety of ways. These range from networks of safe houses in more rural areas of the country; to transition houses that offer shelter, food, emotional support, and access to other services for women and their children; to family resource centers that provide services to a broader range of women with special needs; and to multipurpose shelters, which may serve men as well as women and children (Health and Welfare Canada, 1987).

Although the work of ensuring the availability of a place of safety for any woman in Canada is by no means complete, a second effort to eliminate wife assault has formed, this time with a focus on the perpetrators of the problem—the men who batter. At last count, there are 43 programs across Canada for men who batter

(Health and Welfare Canada, 1986). All groups appear to be based on a group model of therapy (Browning, 1984).

The third wave—attempts to keep wife assault from happening—is only seriously beginning. Ontario has been at the forefront of the domestic violence movement in Canada, and has retained that position with its announcements in September 1986 and April 1987 of substantial funding for preventive counseling, public education, and professional training (Minister of Community and Social Services, September 16, 1986; "Shelters to receive ...", 1987).

This chapter contributes to these preventive efforts by providing an analysis of what is meant by prevention; summarizing the theories of causation of wife assault upon which preventive initiatives might be based; identifying the underlying assumptions of these theories; and specifying their implications for program development. I then outline the primary, secondary, and tertiary preventive efforts that would follow from adopting each of the perspectives on etiology, and summarize what is known empirically about efforts to prevent wife assault to date. I conclude by proposing a model of service that I believe will most effectively meet the goal of reducing both the prevalence and the incidence of wife assault.

WHAT IS PREVENTION?

The literature on prevention distinguishes among primary, secondary, and tertiary interventions (Bloom, 1981; Borkin & Siegel, 1983; Canadian Council on Social Development, 1982; Caplan, 1964; Geismar, 1969; Lorion, 1983). Although there are differences of opinion as to the precise meaning of each of these categories, they can best be understood in terms of their relationship to the incidence or prevalence of a problem. *Incidence* means the number of new cases in a specified period. *Prevalence* means the total number of cases present in the population at a given time. Another way of saying this is that these three types of intervention can best be understood in terms of their desired outcomes. Primary, secondary, and tertiary prevention are defined briefly here, and then discussed in the context of wife assault.

Tertiary prevention, commonly called *rehabilitation* (Bloom, 1981; Borkin & Siegel, 1983; Geismar, 1969) is defined by efforts to reduce the duration of a problem and to minimize the impairment resulting to an individual, couple, family, or community from the disorder. It could also have the goal of achieving a more positive level of functioning than had previously been demonstrated, as with health promotion programs, or some skills development programs. The focus of these interventions is solely on reducing the prevalence of the identified problem.

Secondary prevention is defined variously as treatment (Bloom, 1981), intervention (Borkin & Siegel, 1983), or remediation (Geismar, 1969). These programs also share the goal of decreasing the prevalence of the target problem by reducing its duration or severity, but the interventions are initiated in the early stages of the problem (Geismar, 1969). Crisis intervention for drug abusers or a program for first-time young offenders, for example, would be considered secondary prevention.

Primary prevention, what Bloom (1981) suggested we simply call *prevention*, differs from both secondary and tertiary prevention in that it has as its goal not treatment or rehabilitation but a reduction in the onset of new cases of the identified disorder or problem (Lorion, 1983). Consequently, it has an impact not only on the incidence of a problem, but on its prevalance as well. Theoretically, primary prevention could lead to the elimination of a disorder if preventive efforts were effective, and were sustained over a sufficiently long period of time.

These distinctions might be clearer if they are applied to the services offered to the men, women, and children involved in battering incidents. Groups for men who batter or assertiveness training for women would be examples of tertiary prevention. The goal is to achieve more positive functioning—to increase the man's ability to control his anger or to increase the woman's ability to assert herself. Transition housing, crisis counseling offered to women in shelters, or the interventions of domestic violence teams might be considered secondary prevention. They also have the goal of reducing the prevalence of wife assault, but the focus is on lessening the more immediate effects of a battering incident. Primary prevention, then, would include programs that target high-risk groups like children of abusing couples, teaching boys and girls problem-solving communication and assertiveness skills. The goal would be to help these high-risk children avoid being the primary actors in battering incidents of their own. Broadly focused efforts such as public education programs, sex-role socialization for equality between men and women, or training programs for professionals might also be considered primary prevention.

Bloom (1981) argued that one of the characteristics of primary prevention is that it is based on a theory of causation. An extension of this position would be to suggest that effective program development, whether for primary, secondary, or tertiary prevention, should be based on explicit assumptions about etiology. In the following section, a summary is made of the theories that have been offered in the literature to explain why wife assault occurs, the underlying assumptions identified, and the programming implications discussed.

WHAT CAUSES WIFE ASSAULT?

A variety of theories have been offered to explain why men batter women (Dobash & Dobash, 1979; Dutton, 1983; Gelles & Straus, 1979; Straus, 1973, 1977-1978; Walker, 1979). Almost an equal number of typologies have been developed to group these theories in some meaningful way (Browning, 1984; Gondolf, 1985b; Lystad, 1982; Pahl, 1985; Straus, 1977; Walker, 1984b). For purposes of discussion here, they are categorized as psychological, sociological, or integrated theories.

Psychological Theories

Psychological theories tend to see the functioning of either the husband or the wife as the source of family violence. This might be because they are mentally ill—the husband sadistic, psychopathic, or perhaps brain-damaged (Browning, 1984; Schultz, 1960), and the wife masochistic (Garbarino & Gilliam, 1980; Kleckner, 1978; Lion, 1977; Shainess, 1979; Snell, Rosenwald, & Robey, 1964) or alcoholic. Early family systems theorists like Minuchin (1974) who saw the family as a closed system and therefore failed to take into account social, economic, or political factors might also be included in this category. James and McIntyre (1983) argue that systems theory does not even permit the question of causality to be raised. This is a theory that focuses on problem maintenance, it is suggested, rather than on etiology (Avis, 1988).

Recent work suggests that mental illness can be a factor in wife assault, but that it is no more common among wife abusers than it is in the general population (Pressman, 1984). It is clear that alcohol is a factor in wife assault, with as many as 44% of offenders reported under its influence at the time of the assault (Byles, 1982). It appears that it is not a causal factor, however, as family counseling has proven successful in eliminating violence even when drinking continues (Knowles, 1980). Work by Ganley (1981) also shows that abusers are about evenly divided among four groups: those who abuse only when they are drunk; those who abuse whether they are drunk or sober; those who are social drinkers but who are not drunk when they abuse; and those who never drink.

The underlying assumption of the psychological framework is that wife assault is a private matter, not a public one, and should therefore be dealt with on a case-by-case basis. The political ideology of those accepting this explanation tends to be what George and Wilding (1985) call anti-collectivist, or more commonly, conservative. The primary tenet of this position is that the individual, not the public, is responsible for his or her own well-being. The perception of women's roles that is congruent with this perspective is what Shaevitz (1984) called traditional; that is, women are seen as men's lesser, not their equal. As such, they should accept the direction of their husbands and define their primary role as one of service to their husbands and children. In keeping with the anti-collectivist ideology, which advocates minimal government provision of services, those adopting a psychological explanation of the cause of wife assault would also tend to support a residual perspective of the social service system (Wilensky & Lebeaux, 1965).

With respect to programming, those adopting a psychological explanation for wife abuse would develop preventive strategies that are principally tertiary, with limited secondary interventions. The onus for seeking help would clearly rest with individual men and women. An incremental or laissez-faire approach to planning would be adopted under this theoretical orientation, with new programs being developed on an ad hoc basis when a need for them was perceived in a given agency. Funding for services would be through charitable donations or fee-for-service, except for the police or the courts that would be publicly funded. With the exception of the police and court systems, services would be delivered through the voluntary sector or private practitioners. Therapists involved in a counseling relationship with abusing men or abused women would tend to have a psychoanalytic orientation, or a traditional systems perspective based on the premise that the family is a closed system.

Sociocultural Theories

The second category of theories, the sociocultural, posits that battering behavior is either learned from having experienced violence in one's family of origin, through the general acceptance of violence in our broader culture, or results from a man's need to assert his power or domination over women. Social learning theory suggests that the violent behavior of men against women can be explained by the fact that these men have observed their fathers assaulting their mothers and/or were themselves abused by their parents as children. Thus, they are modeling the behavior of their parents when they batter. Straus, Gelles, and Steinmetz's (1980) work provides support for this theory, showing that 1 in 10 husbands who grew up in violent homes are wife beaters, compared to 1 in 30 who grew up in nonviolent homes.

Walker's (1979, 1984b) work is based on social learning theory as well, but focuses on the experience of women in a battering relationship. She identified what she called "learned helplessness" or the "battered woman syndrome." Women learn helplessness, she said, as a result of repeatedly experiencing beatings for no apparent reason. The unpredictability of the timing and of the precipitators of these events leads a woman to conclude that she cannot control what happens to her. Once she has submitted to this belief, it becomes real in its consequences. That is, even if she is successful in avoiding a battering incident, she cannot believe that this success can be repeated. Like Seligman's (1975) dogs, her motivation to try to help herself is eventually eroded to the point where she can no longer see opportunities to protect herself, even when they are presented. Women are particularly susceptible to learned helplessness in their relationships with men, Walker said, because of their sex-role socialization. Thus, learned helplessness is not a consequence of an individual character flaw, but of a social system that teaches women that they should please their mates rather than meet their own needs, and that they bear primary responsibility for the quality of relationships in family life.

Cultural theory also argues that violent behavior is learned, but emphasizes the legitimation of violence by society in general rather than in the family alone (Breines & Gordon, 1983; Straus, 1977, 1977-1978; Sutton, 1978; Tomes, 1978). Straus (1977) argues that violence is condoned in American culture in such pervasive ways as the death penalty, widespread ownership of handguns and through the media. I would add to this the high level of expenditure on military armaments. It is noteworthy that RAVEN, a men's program in St. Louis, identifies military training as one of the factors contributing to wife abuse (Gondolf, 1985a).

These cultural practices reflect a value system that leads to 20% of Americans agreeing it is acceptable to slap their spouse on appropriate occasions and 90% of parents using spanking as a form of discipline with children (Stark & McEvoy, 1970).

Power-based theories argue that the issue of wife abuse is not merely one of violence, but of power relationships between men and women (Dobash & Dobash, 1979; Gondolf, 1985b; Pressman, 1984). In pre-Christian times, before the role of men in procreation was understood, women were seen as goddesses, possessing the gift of reproducing life. Once man's role was understood, however, Davidson (1977) and Daly (1978) argue that women lost that position of dominance, and matriarchy gave way to patriarchy. Christianity reinforced women's inferiority, they say, with the story of Eve precipitating the fall from grace by tempting Adam to eat the forbidden fruit. Women's lesser status is further reinforced by the many Biblical exhortations for woman to be subject to her husband, and Paul's assertion that woman was made from man, not man from woman. The legal systems in Britain, the United States, and Canada further reinforced women's oppression by enacting laws that permitted a man to physically abuse his wife, provided that the abuse was not too extreme. Dobash and Dobash (1979) have developed this perspective most fully, summarizing their argument by asserting that violence against women is a means of controlling and oppressing them, an extension of patriarchical domination. Advocates of power-based theories differ from those supporting learned behavior theories, then, in that they do not see men's and women's traditional sex-role socialization as something that evolved over time, but rather as a deliberate effort on the part of men to control women.

The underlying assumption of sociocultural theories is that changes can be made in our family and social structures that will reduce, or perhaps eliminate, the incidence of wife assault. Violent behavior has been learned within the family, the theory argues, so families must be supported and strengthened in ways that can eliminate the violence. Society has permitted violence against women through its laws and mores, so society can change these laws and send a new message—that violence is no longer acceptable. Family violence is, therefore, a public issue, not a private matter.

The political ideology of those accepting sociocultural explanations of wife assault would tend to be what George and Wilding (1985) call Fabian socialists, or more commonly, social democrats. This means that they would see structural factors like the socialization process and the distribution of power as primarily responsible for creating the problem of wife assault. Consequently, there is a need for a public or collective commitment to deal with it. One result of that willingness to have government intervene would be greater support for expenditures on services to address the problem of wife assault. Thus, they would tend to support an institutional model of social services (Wilensky & Lebeaux, 1965).

With respect to women's role, those accepting learning theory as the causal explanation would tend to be what Jaggar (1983) called liberal feminists. They would see the roots of women's oppression in sex-role socialization, and freedom from this oppression coming through the repeal of sex-based laws, through the provision of services to women, through public education, and through equality of opportunity for women within our existing economic structure.

Those accepting power-based theories are more likely to be what Jaggar (1983) has called socialist or radical feminists. Although feminists of all persuasions are committed to greater equality between men and women, socialist and radical feminists would support different strategies than liberal feminists. The socialist feminist sees equality being realized by addressing gender differences in a similar way to the liberal feminist, but she also sees a need for class differences to be reduced. These differences are based on an unequal distribution of economic and political power. The radical feminist, by contrast, sees this happening through the development of a woman culture that would be separate from mainstream, patriarchal culture and would permit women finally to exercise control over their own lives. As such, they would tend to advocate an alternate service system, for women only.

Marxist feminists have not been included in this discussion because of the primacy they give to the issue of class (Jaggar, 1983). Rather than supporting any service strategy to deal with an issue like wife assault, they would tend to advocate the support of efforts to eliminate class differences. Once a classless society is achieved, they believe problems such as wife assault would disappear.

Preventive efforts that would follow from adopting a sociocultural explanation of etiology would be tertiary, secondary, and primary. The primary preventive intervention would have two foci. The first would be strengthening high-risk groups such as children from abusive families so that they do not become involved in battering relationships in their families of procreation. The second would be on efforts to socialize boys and girls to more egalitarian sex roles and on advocating structural changes that would promote the equality of women.

Program planning under this perspective would address the problem of wife assault comprehensively or holistically. A full array of services and supports required to reduce wife assault would be identified and put into place over time. Funding for these services would be primarily public with more emphasis on public by those with a socialist than a liberal ideology. Service delivery would also be primarily through the public sector, again with greater emphasis on the public sector by those with a socialist ideology. Those involved in therapeutic relationships with abusing men and women would tend to be psychoeducational, with an emphasis on understanding how gender roles and power differentials between men and women have permitted wife assault to occur.

Integrated Theories

Recently, work in the area of the etiology of family violence has shifted to focus on what might be called an *integrated approach*. A seminal paper by Belsky (1980) suggested that perspectives identifying single factors are inadequate to develop a meaningful understanding of child abuse. He argued, rather, that it is necessary to look at the combined impact of individual developmental factors on the parents and the child (ontogenetic factors); of family functioning (microsystem); of community functioning—including neighbors, and the workplace—(ecosystem); and of the broader culture (macrosystem). Dutton (1983) has applied this analysis to the problem of wife assault.

A similar argument is made in the work of women identifying themselves as feminist therapists who have been struggling with the issue of whether family systems and feminist theory are compatible in the therapeutic context (Avis, 1988; Bograd, 1984; Goldner, 1985a; Hare-Mustin, 1978; Libow, Raskin, & Caust, 1982; Magill, Chapter 4, this volume; Pressman, Chapter 3, this volume). Although a family systems perspective is seen as more useful than the early psychoanalytic models in working with families where wife assault occurs, Bograd (1984) argued that it still contains "subtle but pernicious biases that inadvertently sanction violence against women or that deflect attention away from the social conditions that may engender battering" (p.560).

Specific concerns with the systems perspective identified by feminists include the conceptualization of causality (Bograd, 1984; Libow et al., 1982; Magill, Chapter 4, this volume; Pressman, Chapter 3, this volume); the context seen as pertinent in dealing with a problem (Bograd, 1984; Hare-Mustin, 1978; Libow et al., 1982; Magill, Chapter 4, this volume); the therapist's use of self (Libow et al., 1982; Pressman, Chapter 3, this volume); and the strategies seen as appropriate for effecting change (Libow et al., 1982; Pressman, Chapter 3, this volume). A brief elaboration of these points is set out here. For a more detailed discussion, see either chapter 4 by Magill or chapter 3 by Pressman earlier in this book.

The systems perspective is based on a concept of circular causality that defines each action as both being caused by other actions or events and, in turn, causing some other action or effect. Cause really becomes a meaningless term, then, in the sense that cause and effect are inseparable (Libow et al., 1982). A male's violent behavior is not seen as being explained by factors within the family but is a consequence or symptom of the functioning within the family system. The feminist therapist, by contrast, has a more traditional, linear concept of causality (Libow et al., 1982). Violent behavior is seen as resulting not only from relations within the family, but from factors that are temporally prior to its formation, like the gender roles to which partners were socialized and power inequalities that exist between men and women in patriarchal societies.

The context on which one focuses from a systems perspective is the microsystem of the family. Feminist therapists would also take into consideration factors associated with the client's community and broader culture. The target of change for the family systems therapist, consequently, is the pattern of interaction between the couple. The feminist therapist would be actively involved in consciousness-raising and in promoting social change as well.

The emphasis of the family systems therapist is on changing behaviors in either the male or female partner that permit violence to erupt. In contrast, the feminist therapist attempts to promote insight or understanding of the attitudes and beliefs that give rise to the violent episodes thereby bringing them to an end. With respect to use of self, the family therapist assumes the traditional role of expert, retaining a certain distance from and superiority to the client. The feminist therapist approaches the therapeutic relationship as an equal, and will commonly reveal personal experiences as a means of promoting an egalitarian relationship.

An extension of one's orientation to use of self is the therapist determining which strategies are seen as appropriate for effecting change. The family systems therapist may use paradoxical injunction, behavioral prescription, task assignment, positioning, structural rearrangement, and reframing (Libow et al., 1982). These strategies may involve manipulation of the family rather than collaboration with them. The feminist therapist by comparison, emphasizes direct, open communication. She rejects the use of manipulation or indirect suggestion.

The underlying assumption of the integrated theories is that wife assault is a complex issue that can only be explained by looking at a combination of psychological, sociological, political, and economic factors. The political ideology of those supporting this explanation of the cause of wife assault might be either George and Wilding's (1985) reluctant collectivist or their Fabian socialist. This means that they would see both society and the individual as having some responsibility for the creation and maintenance of the problem of wife assault. Consequently, they would support public funding of programs in this area, although less enthusiastically than those accepting sociocultural explanations. They would support the provision of some part of the services through the private nonprofit (voluntary) sector and the private for-profit sector as well. The model of social services consistent with this perspective, then, would also be institutional (Wilensky & Lebeaux, 1965), although less completely so than with those accepting sociocultural theories of etiology.

Those accepting an integrated theoretical explanation of the causes of wife assault are almost certainly feminists. To accept the premise that relationships between men and women must become more egalitarian is to accept the basic premise of feminism. Radical feminists would be likely to emphasize consciousness-raising through a neutral support group model and an alternate system for delivery of service. Socialist feminists would likely have a similar emphasis on consciousness-raising, although they would be more likely to accept provision of services through the established service delivery system than radical feminists. They would also be concerned about economic issues like pay equity that have an impact on maintaining class differences. Liberal feminists might start their own voluntary organizations, but would be likely to see themselves a part of other existing service delivery systems. Liberal feminists might also use consciousness-raising groups. In addition, they might do consciousness-raising on a one-to-one basis or use approaches in working with families where wife assault has occurred that are based on psychodynamic or family systems theories where the family is seen as an open system.

Those supporting an integrated approach to understanding the cause of wife assault would see the need for a comprehensive array of services to meet the needs of the women, men and children involved in this violence. They would therefore provide primary, secondary, and tertiary services, with a stronger emphasis on the tertiary than those accepting sociocultural explanations of wife assault.

Summary

Table 10.1 summarizes three groups of theories of wife assault which have been identified in this section; those seeing the source of the problem in psychological factors, those seeing it in sociocultural factors, and those seeing it in a combination of the two. These theoretical perspectives have been summarized, the underlying assumptions identified, and the implications for programming of adopting each of the three theories spelled out. In the section that follows, I set out the primary, secondary, and tertiary prevention interventions that would be part of a service delivery system based on each of these orientations.

PREVENTIVE STRATEGIES SUPPORTED
BY EACH THEORY OF CAUSATION

Wife assault is a complex problem, touching on at least 11 areas of service delivery: housing, counseling, child care, social assistance, policing, the courts, medical care, education, job retraining, research, and social action. The recent policy initiatives in Ontario, for instance, involve nine ministries. Table 10.2 summarizes the preventive strategies supported by each of the theories of causation, using the service delivery areas mentioned earlier for purposes of analyses.

Psychological Theories

Under psychological theories of causation, services for assaulted women, their children and their partners would be minimal. Individual counseling would be available and would tend to be based on a psychoanalytic perspective. If couple counseling were done, it would be based on the premise that the family is a closed system. Advocacy services would be unlikely. Police would intervene in only the most severe cases of assault, and would seldom lay charges, even when the attack was sufficient to hospitalize a woman. In those cases where charges were laid by the spouse or the police, lawyers, and judges would be reluctant to get involved in family affairs. Legal aid would be available, but few lawyers would participate because of the low fee schedule.

Crisis shelter would consist of multipurpose emergency housing that would accommodate men and women, and would lack support services such as crisis

TABLE 10.1
Programming Implications of Theories of Causation

Theory of Causation	Concept of Service Delivery System	Programming Issues				
		Planning Approach	Preventive Strategies	Funding	Service Delivery Sector	Therapeutic Orientation of Counselors
Psychological	Residual	Incremental	Tertiary, some secondary	Private: Fee-for-service or charitable donations except for police and courts	Voluntary, private practice	Psychoanalytic or traditional family systems (family a system)
Sociocultural	Institutional	Comprehensive – Equality for women	Tertiary, secondary, primary – High-risk groups; Structural changes	Public	Public	Feminist-consciousness raising, primarily through mutual support groups
Integrated	Social Developmental	Comprehensive – Wife assault in particular, but equality for women more generally	Tertiary, secondary, primary – High-risk groups; Structural changes	Public/private mix	Voluntary, private practice, public	Feminist-consciousness raising – mutual support group; Psychodynamic theories; Family systems (family an open system)

TABLE 10.2

Preventive Strategies Supported by Each of the Theories of Causation

Theory of Causation	Preventive Strategies		
	Primary	*Secondary*	*Tertiary*
Psychological	Education: Responsibility of individual or family; no public education programs; no professional training in family violence	Police: Intervene only in most severe cases; seldom lay charges; not trained in how to handle domestic violence teams	Counseling: Individual counseling within a psychoanalytic practice framework; couple counseling from early systems perspective; advocacy services unlikely
	Research: Public funding not available	Courts: Judges reluctant to intervene in family affairs; legal aid available, but limited number of lawyers participate; cases heard in Family Court	Housing: Second-stage housing not available; affordable, accessible housing not available
	Social action: Collective efforts to effect change unlikely	Housing: Crisis shelters not available; multipurpose emergency housing may exist, but without supports	Child care: Affordable, accessible child care not available
		Medical Care: Staff not trained; no protocol for dealing with wife assault; recording inadequate	Social assistance: Benefit levels inadequate; stigma associated with receiving benefits
			Retraining: Not available through public sector

Socio-cultural	Education: Public responsibility; emphasis on high risk groups; involvement in general education efforts to help boys and girls learn more egalitarian sexroles; public education program re availability of services and laws respecting wife assault; empowerment of women through assertiveness training, communication skills; training program for all involved with wife assault	Police: Intervene in all cases of wife assault; charges laid in all cases where there is probable cause; well-trained on issue of wife assault; domestic violence teams on every force	Counseling: Feminist counseling for women; consciousness-raising groups, mutual support groups; advocacy services; ongoing treatment for children and men
	Research: Funding available; for work in areas of treatment, rehabilitation and policy; evaluation of programs and policies to determine whether they are reducing wife assault	Courts: Mandatory treatment for all wife abusers; judges well-trained; legal aid available and most lawyers participate; all cases heard in Criminal Court	Housing: Second-stage housing available; geared-to-income housing available on a priority basis
		Housing: Crisis shelters in numbers that reflect the problem; full range of support services including child care, crisis counseling and therapeutic programming for children	Child care: Accessible, affordable child care available on a priority basis to assaulted women
	Social action: Use of lobby groups like National Action Committee on the Status of Women to effect changes in policies, procedures and laws having a negative effect on assaulted women; those seeing power differences between men and women as key to inequality would advocate social and economic changes to reduce these inequalities	Medical care: Staff well-trained on issue of wife assault; protocol for treatment available; recording sufficiently detailed and complete to be effective in court hearings	Social assistance: Benefit levels adequate; minimal stigma associated with receiving benefits
			Retraining: Good access to retraining programs; well-paying, nontraditional jobs emphasized

counseling or child care. Medical staff would not know how to support the abused woman or to document her injuries in a way that would be helpful in court. Should a woman decide to separate from her partner, she would find little affordable housing, limited subsidized day-care spaces, inadequate social assistance benefits, and limited publicly funded retraining opportunities. There would be few professional training or public education programs on family violence. Little would be known about the prevalence of wife assault, its etiology or how to treat it, because public funding would be limited for research in this area. Finally, there would be no organized efforts to bring about changes that would better meet the needs of women. In summary, the service delivery system under this perspective is what has existed in Canada historically and continues to exist in many parts of the country.

Sociocultural Theories

A more complete service delivery system would exist than that described under the psychological theories to meet the assumptions of the sociocultural model, with a broad range of tertiary, secondary, and primary services being offered. Long-term (tertiary) counseling would be available for women, children, and men involved in battering relationships with an emphasis on helping them understand gender-role socialization and how it has promoted women's inequality. For women and men, this insight takes place in segregated consciousness-raising groups. For women, these might be supplemented by assertiveness training, conflict resolution, and mutual support groups. For men, they might be supplemented by anger management and conflict resolution skills. Consciousness-raising would also be important for children, who are socialized to gender roles daily as they observe men and women, particularly their parents, interact. They also might profit from developing their conflict resolution skills. Counselors involved in these programs would have a strong commitment to advocating for their clients.

In the area of secondary preventive strategies, police would be well-trained with respect to family violence, domestic violence teams would be common, and policy would direct them to lay charges against batterers. When there was probable cause, and they would have indepth training in this, they would lay charges. Judges and lawyers would also be well-trained with respect to wife assault. Judges would generally require mandatory treatment for batterers. Legal Aid would be available to cover a woman's legal costs, and most lawyers would accept legal aid clients.

Crisis shelters for battered women would exist in most communities and would be funded sufficiently to provide a full range of support services, including child care, crisis counseling, and ongoing support services for the battered woman and her children. Medical staff would be trained in issues of family violence and would have a well-developed protocol for use with battered women that would result in records useful in court proceedings. Women deciding to separate from their partners would find that they had access to subsidized housing and day care. Social assistance benefit levels would be adequate and the stigma associated with being a welfare client would be less than at present. Retraining opportunities would be available for women and would tend to emphasize well-paying jobs, some of which would be nontraditional.

The service delivery system under the sociocultural perspective would differ greatly from that under the psychological perspective in that there would be substantial resources invested in prevention. The principal focus of these efforts would be on children identified as high risk by virtue of being raised in a family where wife or child abuse occurred and on empowering women. Programming goals would include improving problem-solving skills, communication skills, and assertiveness for men and women, boys and girls, and anger control and affective expression for men and boys. A widespread public education program would make people aware of the incidence of wife assault, services available for those assaulted and their assaulters, and send a clear message that wife assault would not be tolerated. Continuing in the preventive vein, public research monies would be available, and there would evolve a reasonable understanding of the prevalence and etiology of wife assault. There would be a commitment to evaluating program outcomes, though the funding implications may mean that sufficient resources are not allocated to do the job thoroughly.

Finally, collective action would be taken to effect changes in laws, policies, or procedures that negatively affect assaulted women. A women's lobby group such as the National Action Committee on the Status of Women might be used, or a special purpose group might be organized with a focus on wife assault or family violence.

Integrated Theories

The final service delivery model described is based on the belief that wife assault is a complex issue that can only be explained by looking at a combination of psychological, sociological, political, and economic factors. It is a synthesis of the psychological and sociocultural theories. As such, it is very similar to the sociocultural model, differing primarily in the type of tertiary counseling services that would be provided. Although the sociocultural theories would lead one to an emphasis on consciousness raising, asertiveness training, and conflictresolution, the integrated approach would add to these a consideration of the factors in the development of both male and female partners, and in their relationship that have resulted in the explosion of violence. This approach would also place greater emphasis on dealing with the trauma to a woman who has been assaulted (Pressman, chapter 3, this volume).

In the area of primary and secondary prevention, the services provided would be similar to those supported under the sociocultural model. Any difference in the two would be in degree of commitment to government intervention on this issue, with those adopting a sociocultural perspective more fully committed to public funding.

Summary

Three service delivery models have been outlined and are summarized in Tables 10.1 - 10.4, one based on a psychological explanation of wife assault, the second on a sociocultural explanation, and the third on an integration of these two theories. The intent of this section was to demonstrate that the theory of causation that one adopts leads to support for a different package of primary, secondary, and tertiary services for dealing with the problem of wife assault. The theory one chooses is related to one's political ideology, which has implications for programming issues not only in the therapeutic context, but in the area of instrumental assistance as well. Although it is sometimes thought that ideology is the most compelling determinant in choosing a theoretical approach, one must take into account also what is known empirically about the outcomes or effects of the services that are being offered. Consequently, when developing a model for prevention of wife assault in the next section, a summary is made of the limited number of empirical findings that are as yet available on the impact of services to violent families.

WHAT DO WE KNOW EMPIRICALLY
ABOUT PREVENTING WIFE ASSAULT?

Given that we knew little about the prevalence or etiology of wife assault until recently, it should not be surprising that we are only now beginning to learn about the outcomes or effects of the services we offer to battered women, their children and their partners. A review of the literature revealed only five studies that might be considered evaluative. One of these is the recent survey of shelter workers by Linda MacLeod (1987), a second is a follow-up study of women who had used a shelter (Regina Women's Transition Society, 1984), and the last three are studies of the effects of police-charging policies (Burris & Jaffee, 1983; Jaffee, Wolfe, Telford, & Austin, 1986; Sherman & Berk, 1984a&b). Although limited in number, these studies provide us with important information for program development

First , they tell us that shelters are being used. In 1985, 3,000 women in Canada were housed for one or more nights in order to escape abuse. About an equal number were turned away which suggests that we still do not have enough beds to meet the need (MacLeod, 1987).

Second, they tell us that even though a woman has been beaten by a man, she may want to continue the relationship. Estimates are that 33% (Regina Women's Transition Society, 1984) to 50% (Katz, 1986) of women return to their partners. These data support the need for men's services. Ganley (1981) recommended that these be provided through groups, and that they be court-ordered, as abusing men

TABLE 10.3
Proposed Model of Prevention

Theory of Causation	Preventive Strategies		
	Primary	*Secondary*	*Tertiary*
Integrated	Education: Public responsibility; joint emphasis on high risk groups and employment of women; training programs for all professionals with respect to wife assault and the promotion of more egalitarian treatment of women Research: Funding available; for work in areas of treatment, rehabilitation and policy; evaluation of programs and policies to determine whether they are reducing wife assault Social action: Use of lobby groups like National Action Committee on the Status of Women to effect changes in policies, procedure and laws having a negative effect on assaulted women; those seeing power differences between men and women as key to inequality would advocate social and economic changes to reduce these inequalities	Police: Intervene in all cases of wife assault reported; lay charges in all cases; well-trained on issues of wife assault; domestic violence team on every force Courts: Mandatory counseling for wife abusers; judges well-trained; legal aid available and most lawyers participate; all cases heard in Criminal Court Housing: Crisis shelters available in numbers that reflect problem; accessible; full range of support services e.g. child care, crisis counseling, advocacy services Medical care: Staff well-trained on issues of wife assault; protocol for treatment available; recording sufficiently complete and detailed to be effective in court hearings	Counseling: Systems-based feminist counseling for men, women and children; self-help support groups; advocacy services for all women Housing: Second-stage housing available; geared-to-income housing available on a priority basis Child care: Accessible, affordable child care available; on a priority basis to assaulted women. Social assistance: Benefit levels adequate; minimal stigma associated with receipt of benefits Retraining: Good access to retraining programs; well-paying, nontraditional jobs emphasized

often do not see anything wrong with their behavior. Consequently, they are likely to drop out of a program, or never get to it, unless ordered by the court.

Third, they remind us that children are involved in family violence too, sometimes as witnesses and sometimes as victims (MacLeod, 1987; Regina Women's Transition Society, 1984). In 1985, 55,000 children were cared for in shelters, half of them under the age of 5 (MacLeod, 1987). They also have needs that should be met by programming in the shelter and on an ongoing basis if the cycle of violence is to be ended. Recent policy in Ontario recognizes this and explicitly provides funding for children's counseling in shelters.

Fourth, only a small percentage of battered women will ever use a shelter. One estimate is that as few as 11% use crisis housing (Katz, 1986). The remainder need information, referral, counseling, and accompaniment to court. This supports the need for information and advocacy services for battered women, whether they make use of shelters or not.

Fifth, there is evidence that if police lay charges against abusers they are less likely to repeat the violence than if they are offered advice or separated from their partners (Burris & Jaffee, 1983; Jaffee, Wolfe, Telford, & Austin, 1986; Sherman & Berk, 1984a&b). Further, charges are less likely to be withdrawn if they are laid by police, and wife assault victims report greater satisfaction with police intervention when they charge (Jaffee, Wolfe, Telford, & Austin, 1986). These data clearly support a policy of police charging.

Although the studies cited here are scanty, they are a beginning. They point to a number of important questions which need to be addressed in future research. Perhaps chief among them is which services for men are effective in reducing violence. If women continue to live with men who have assaulted them, it is critical that we identify ways to work with men to bring wife assault to an end. One of the current developments that looks promising is groups for men. It will be important to determine whether they are effective by themselves or only in conjunction with police laying of charges and mandatory group attendance. It will also be important to determine what the focus of these groups should be: anger control, attitudes toward women, or conflict resolution, for instance. A further area that is critical for future research is children's programming. At this time, we do not know what type of programming is being done for children or which approaches are most effective with different age and gender groups. Nor do we know if the approaches to be used should differ if the child was an observer only or a victim of violence him or herself. We also lack evidence on the effectiveness of public education programs. These programs are difficult to evaluate, because an effective program may actually result in an increase in the reported incidence of violence according to measures like number of domestic calls for police. Surveys that focused on attitudes toward the acceptance of violence may be useful in this endeavor. Finally, more research might be done on the effects of police charging. Follow-ups beyond the 6-month period would be useful to determine how long the apparent deterrent effect lasts.

A PROPOSED MODEL OF PREVENTION

Many questions remain unanswered as to whether programs currently being offered to deal with the problem of wife assault are having their intended effects. In spite of these unanswered questions, services must continue to be delivered to families where battering occurs. In this section, I suggest seven principles, three based on ideology and four on research findings, that I believe should provide the foundation for a model of service with this population. The assumption underlying all of these principles is that the goal of an effective model of service must be to reduce the incidence and prevalence of wife assault; that is, it must place a priority on primary prevention.

The ideologically based principles are:

1. Violence is unacceptable as a way of expressing oneself within the family.
2. Women are equal to men and have a right to be treated with the same respect and consideration given to men.
3. We have a collective, or public, responsibility to end family violence.

The empirically based principles are:

1. A model of service must recognize that a significant proportion of women will continue their relationships with men who have battered them.
2. A model of service must recognize that children are involved in significant numbers of these relationships and are themselves affected by the violence either directly or as observers.
3. Information and support service must be provided for the great majority of women who are assaulted yet never use the services of a shelter.
4. The policy of police charging should be more rigorously enforced in light of its apparent effect on reducing the incidence of recidivism among men who abuse.

As Canadians, we have already made a commitment to each of the three value-based principles identified for this model. The Solicitor General of Canada has directed Chiefs of Police to instruct their officers to lay charges against men who assault (MacLeod, 1987). The Charter of Rights and Freedoms, passed in April 1982, asserts more clearly than the previous Human Rights Code that women are to be treated as men's equals. To a greater extent in some provinces than in others, monies are now being spent on services that address the problem of wife assault. In summary, there appears to be the political will to end wife assault, and more generally, family violence. That is, we appear to have made a collective or public commitment to the ideological principles outlined here, even if each one of us has not made the commitment individually.

A review of the causal theories suggests that either the sociocultural or the integrated theories, but not the psychological, would be compatible with these principles. What of the empirically based principles then? Again, both the sociocultural and integrated theories generate service models that recognize that large numbers of women continue in their relationships with men who batter them, that children are involved in the violence, that many women are in need of information and support who do not use shelters and that the policy of police charging needs to be enforced more rigorously.

The integrated approach, with its incorporation of family systems theory, adds one piece that the sociocultural does not, however. It permits the therapist not only to work with the husband and the wife separately, but also to look at the elements of their relationship which may have contributed to the violence. As Magill (chapter 4, this volume) notes, to merge a commitment to feminist principles of equality and a conviction that sociocultural factors are the root cause of family violence with an analysis of the couple's relationship is to present oneself with certain contradictions or conflicts. Nonetheless, the insights to be gained by both therapist and client argue for its use, after the male and female have worked on the problem separately, as Pressman (chapter 3, this volume) suggests.

Summary

The question I posed in beginning work on this chapter was "What do we know about preventing wife assault?" A review of the literature shows that our knowledge of the etiology of the problem is still very much in the developmental stage, though by now one can reasonably classify the theories into one of three categories: the psychological, the sociocultural, and the integrated. Empirical knowledge about which policies or programs appear to reduce the incidence or prevalence of the problem is also limited. Given this relatively preliminary state of knowledge, it may appear early to propose models of service that focus on prevention. Nonetheless, we are daily faced with the challenge of providing support to women, men and children who are caught in the horror of family violence. It therefore seems reasonable to develop services based on a model that takes advantage of what we do now know, theoretically and empirically, not withstanding the need to refine the model as our understanding of the problem increases.

11

Community Development Principles and Helping Battered Women: A Summary Chapter

Gary Cameron
Wilfrid Laurier University

This book includes chapters that were solicited in order to provide an examination of the potential and the limitations of a variety of helping strategies with battered women, their children, and their assailants. Our basic objective was to expand our concept of helping in these situations of family violence. We were not only interested in an assessment of each method of intervention, but also in a consideration of how these different approaches might be used to complement each other. In order to give a focus and to set limits on our project, a decision was made to concentrate on direct interventions with battered women, their children and their batterers. As a consequence of this choice, discussions of program development, administration, social policies, and so on were not emphasized.

In the introductory chapter to this volume, Barbara Pressman and Michael Rothery highlighted the major clinical and treatment issues emanating from the chosen chapters. In this concluding chapter, the general principles of community development are used as a perspective (Nadler, Hackman, & Lawler, 1979) or a conceptual lens (Allison, 1971) to reconsider the potential of the interventions discussed by the chapter authors. This application of the community development perspective promises to be of interest, if for no other reason than it has been substantially absent from these previous deliberations.

The intent, and hopefully the reality, of this exercise is not to criticize the work of the other contributors to the volume. Rather, the community development framework is used in an effort to complement their efforts and to point out the major questions that arise when this particular perspective is considered relevant to the problems of battered women and their families.

The emphasis in this chapter is on extrapolating some of the less evident community development issues emanating from this volume. As a result, the more straightforward observations such as the need for more resources, for an expanded repertoire of services, for better planning and coordination, for improved social policies are not considered. In addition, our analysis concentrates on the contributions that application of community development principles can make to understanding and developing face-to-face helping strategies with battered women and their families.

AN OVERVIEW OF COMMUNITY
DEVELOPMENT PRINCIPLES

This book has described situations where concerns about a lack of economic and social resources, disenfranchisement, blocked life opportunities, and active oppression are shared by many women. As presented, such concerns do not seem to be fundamentally different from those experienced by other groups of users of social services—for example: poor single mothers on welfare, child welfare families, Canadian Indians living on reserves, and physically handicapped individuals. Community development purports to offer particular insights into helping under such circumstances.

A complete discussion of the strengths and weaknesses of a community development approach to helping is too much to attempt in a single chapter. It is evident that community development is not without its critics and it has its own challenges to overcome (Burghardt, 1982; Cameron, 1985; Chekki, 1979; Head, 1979; Roberts, 1979). Notwithstanding these criticisms, a number of the major principles guiding community development interventions have been identified below as a perspective for re-examining helping battered women and their families:

- When working with an actual or potential community of people, it is essential to pay attention to the commonalities in their lives and to foster actions that build on these shared experiences.

- When a large number of users of social services share common problems, an emphasis on individual or case approaches to helping risks blaming the victim (Ryan, 1976) by the implicit or explicit message that such difficulties can be overcome by a more competent performance by the person(s) experiencing them.

- Successful social involvements are essential to our ongoing well-being and to the development of a positive social identity (Brown, 1986; Cameron, in prep; McCall & Simmons, 1966).

- Lack of access to basic economic and social resources is an important problem for many users of social services. With access to adequate economic and social resources, most people cope adequately with their own problems (Cloward & Piven, 1977; Rappaport, 1977).

- People need to become subjects in their own lives. They need to develop an understanding of their own world and to be proactive in dealing with it. People need to see themselves as competent in important areas of their own environment in order to maintain a positive concept of themselves (Bronfenbrenner, 1979; Friere, 1981).

- People learn by doing for themselves and by working with others. Nonreciprocal services do not develop esteem; they are more likely to rob the recipient of dignity. Helping the victimized and the disenfranchised requires assisting them to build their own power (Alinsky, 1971; Friere, 1981; McKnight, 1977; Withorn, 1984).

- In every actual or potential community of disenfranchised people, there exists untapped potential for leadership and for administering their own affairs. Helping strategies should develop these abilities.

- Collective responses—networks, mutual aid organizations, membership organizations, social action organizations—are essential components of overcoming the inferiorization (Adam, 1978) of a community of people.

- Positions of privilege and power are seldom, if ever, willingly given up. This is as true for professional helpers as for any other group enjoying their relative advantages (Alinsky, 1971; Cameron, 1985).

- When people are the victims of shared injustices and active discrimination, explicit discussion of these issues has to be a fundamental component of the helping process (Adam, 1978; Cameron, 1985; Friere, 1981).

- The concrete circumstances of oppression have to be changed. Oppressors cannot be left unhampered to continue to enjoy their privileges (Adam, 1978; Cameron, 1985; Withorn, 1984).

With this collection of community development principles as a guide, it is relatively easy to abstract a number of issues from the discussions in this volume. This exercise allows us to highlight concerns that were not previously given priority.

POLITICAL ANALYSIS AND HELPING
BATTERED WOMEN

For many of these authors, it is axiomatic that the assault of women cannot be properly understood only as an individual or a family problem. Rather, they argue that this assault must be seen within the context of social norms that condone such controlling violence and the relative powerlessness of women both in the home and in our major societal institutions. The underlying thesis is that social and political arrangements clearly advantage men at the expense of women and these conditions must be changed if the same exploitive patterns are not to continue (see the chapters by McDonald, Palmer & Brown, Pressman, and Westhues in this volume). It follows from this political analysis that the development of an understanding of these discriminatory practices should be a conscious goal of helping strategies with battered women—whenever possible. In addition, interventions with assaulted women need to avoid explicitly or implicitly blaming the victims of violence for predicaments that are not of their own making.

From a community development perspective, two issues emerge from this analysis. First, given the backgrounds of the helpers in the service networks to battered women and their families, how open will such helpers be to the introduction of explicit political content in their work with clients? There is evidence (see McDonald, chapter 8, this volume) that the influence of feminist political analysis over services to battered women is waning with the increase in the number of professionals working in this network. It may be that the dominant professional paradigms and feminist political explanations are not compatible.

Several years ago, one of my graduate students (McCafferty, 1983) investigated the attitudes of 45 graduate clinical social work students toward the principles of feminist therapy. She asked these students to analyze a number of case scenarios—each emphasizing different precepts of feminist therapy—and to propose appropriate interventions. Of her respondents, 80% described themselves as strong or moderate supporters of feminism. When the scenarios included items related to personal feelings or interpersonal dynamics, these were consistently identified and responded to by a large majority of participants. Items related to person–environment relations were addressed by between 40% to 59% of the students. However, when the items required that an explicit connection be made between the personal experiences of individual women and the circumstances of women in general, they were identified by between 0% to 19% of respondents. Indeed, over 60% of these graduate social work students expressed strong reservations about linking the problems presented by individual women to broader societal conditions. Many considered this to be an avoidance of the real issues for these women and their families. Apparently, these fledgling professional social workers had already acquired a strong bias against a political approach to helping.

A second question is whether the therapy and service approaches stressed in this volume are the most appropriate vehicles for developing a shared understanding of the reasons for the assault of women. If the development of an analysis of this broader context is important for battered women, then many of these authors may be ignoring the structural limits to the helping strategies they are proposing. Notwithstanding the stated clinical objective of empowering clients, collective and mutual aid approaches present greater possibilities for change than individual, family or group therapies if increased political understanding and empowerment of women are the goals. Although good therapy and involvement in collective actions are not mutually exclusive, a community development analysis would suggest that exclusive reliance on service and therapy—even feminist therapy— risks blaming the victim by pointing to personal change as the key to future success. By implication, failure to thrive would be because the person has not developed the understanding and the abilities to do so.

THE NEED TO EMPOWER WOMEN

Explicit in the feminist analysis of assault is the need to redress power imbalances between men and women both within families and in larger institutions (see chapters by McDonald, Pressman, and Westhues in this volume). Women have to gain power and men need to learn, or be obliged, to share power. Once again, from a community development perspective, the approaches to helping emphasized in this volume do not lend themselves easily to this kind of empowerment.

Empowerment will come more readily from joining together with similar others and by engaging in a collective process of reflection and action. Adam (1978), based on a study of the process of escape from inferiorization of several stigmatized populations, identified a number of common features central to this process of empowerment:

- the injustice of existing circumstances and the treatment of the inferiorized by the outside dominant groups has to be denounced;

- the inferiorized have to begin to see the commonalities in their circumstances and to think of themselves as an identifiable minority;

- the inferiorized have to create some social space for themselves, within which they can enjoy acceptance, intimacy, relative security and where they can begin to exercise control and freedom of action;

- existing realities have to be evaluated by the inferiorized and counterinterpretations of these realities have to be developed and disseminated among the inferiorized and to members of the broader community;

- everyday realities and patterns of relating to the dominating outsiders— including professional service providers—have to be challenged and new, more self-affirming ways of acting encouraged;

- new patterns of coping with a hostile environment have to be created and shared and, whenever possible, efforts made to change conditions in the broader environment.

Arguably, many of the patterns identified by Adam are found within the women's movement and are not reasonably considered the most immediate concerns for those working directly with battered women and their families. However, a community developer might ask what are the standard operating procedures for connecting those battered women who are willing with this broader movement or for connecting them with each other? For example, in organizing the Family Violence and Family Neglect Conference that preceded this book, we wanted to include program examples of community support groups for battered women. Although we made inquiries across the service network in Ontario, we were unsuccessful in locating examples of this helping strategy and it was not included in our conference.

As mentioned previously, there is a suggestion in this volume that the feminist issues discussed in this section are more clearly associated with an earlier—and less mature?—phase in the development of the service network for battered women and their families (McDonald, chapter 8, this volume). Does this mean that the issues of political analysis and empowerment are not as relevant concerns as they once were? What is the relationship between the increased bureaucratization and professionalization of the service network and the empowerment of women? Will political considerations inevitably be shunted aside? Will the individualized service and therapy strategies for helping battered women and their families inevitably become relatively indistinguishable from those in other established social service sectors?

EQUALITY AND RECIPROCITY
IN THE HELPING RELATIONSHIPS

Feminist therapists criticize traditional methods of therapy on the grounds that they reinforce the dominant position of the therapist in the helping relationships. They argue that the therapeutic relationship must be substantially more equal and reciprocal if women are to be effectively empowered (Greenspan, 1983; Pressman, 1984; Pressman, chapter 3, this volume) Using the perspective of community development, it seems that, even in feminist therapy, the power equation remains strongly biased in favor of the professional and the boundaries between who is helping and who needs help are clearly maintained.

Equality and reciprocity are typically found in relationships between people of similar status. Having access to stable, multidimensional, and reciprocal relationships has been linked empirically and theoretically with an improved ability to cope with a variety of problems and to the development of a positive social identity (Adam, 1978; Bronfenbrenner, 1979; Brown, 1986; Cameron, in prep; McCall & Simmons, 1966). Facilitating personal contact and mutual aid between battered women and involving them in new social roles, networks, and support groups, in addition to therapy, all seem to be practical methods of increasing the levels of equality and reciprocity in helping relationships.

ENVIRONMENTAL STRESS AND ACCESS
TO LIFE OPPORTUNITIES

MacLeod (1987), in her study of Canadian Transition Houses, found that a very substantial majority of the women using these shelters were poor with unstable incomes, had little formal education, and had limited job experience. McDonald (chapters 7 & 8, this volume) highlights the numerous environmental obstacles confronting many women leaving a violent relationship—social isolation, limited revenue, limited affordable housing, no access to decent child care. In addition, the clear link between the high rate of marriage breakdown and the feminization of poverty has been described in recent research (National Council of Welfare, 1988). Palmer and Brown (chapter 5, this volume) review the research evidence demonstrating the connections between low-income, unemployment, low socio-economic status, other failures in managing the social environment and higher rates of domestic violence. Moore and his colleagues (chapter 6, this volume) comment on the importance of external support systems and successful social role performances to overcoming the negative repercussions from family violence.

Notwithstanding the aforementioned, a community development perspective would underline how little attention is paid in this volume to such environmental factors, either as explanations of wife assault or in the approaches proposed to helping battered women and their families. This population shares many environmental characteristics with many other consumer groups in the social services. There is a good deal of evidence that service and treatment strategies **alone** do not produce substantial and enduring changes in these multiproblem situations (Cameron, in prep; Rothery, in prep). Under these circumstances, the development of service packages (Whittaker, 1983), and the joining of professional and informal helping strategies, have often produced superior outcomes (Berkeley Planning Associates, 1977; Edmunson, Bedel, & Gordon, 1984; Froland, Pancoast, Chapman, & Kimboko, 1981; Giarretto, 1982; Lieber & Baker, 1977; Rothery & Cameron, 1985; Videka-Sherman, 1985; Wahler, 1983). There are no self-evident reasons why the prescription should be different for battered women and their families.

Access to ongoing supportive relationships and to adequate economic resources are consistently among the best statistical predictors of successful coping with a range of everyday problems and the prevention of institutionalization for adults and children (Cameron, in prep; Cohen & Wills, 1985; Edmunson et al., 1984;

Garbarino, 1977; Snider & Skoretz, 1983). Community development proposes a range of interventions that promise access to a range of social resources relevant to survival in the community and to the construction of new social identities—both major concerns for many battered women and their children.

THE EMERGING DOMINANCE
OF PROFESSIONAL HELPERS

McDonald (chapter 8, this volume) documents the clear trend toward professionalism in transition houses across Canada. Many of the other authors in this book emphasize interventions that require highly trained helpers (Magill; Moore et al.; Palmer & Brown; Pressman, this volume). Without denigrating the value of these involvements with professionals, this perhaps irreversible trend raises several disquieting questions:

- Can an emphasis on feminist and political analyses be sustained?

- Will linkages to the broader women's movement be developed and maintained?

- Will helping strategies that are not individualized and short-term be acceptable?

- Will environmental issues be accorded important consideration in comparison with concerns with intra-personal and family dynamics?

If the experiences from other social service sectors is germane, then the answer to each of the above questions may not be encouraging—either from a feminist or a community development perspective.

CONCLUSIONS

In this summary chapter, a community development perspective was used to review the volume's discussions of helping battered women and their families. Our hope was that this analysis would be consistent with the theme of expanding our concept of helping that provided the initial motivation for this book. In fact, the exercise did point to a number of service and support issues not emphasized elsewhere in the volume:

- the lack of attention paid to informal helping and to community development approaches with this population;

- the apparent contradiction among concerns with empowerment, feminist political analysis, consciousness-raising and many of the service/therapy strategies proposed;

- the relative lack of importance placed on environmental factors in explaining and in designing interventions in situations of wife battering.

Tremendous progress has been made in publicizing and confronting violence toward women over the past decade. These successes have been accompanied by increased public funding of services, larger formal service organizations, and an influx of professionals into important positions. Much has been gained, but perhaps not without cost.

Our wish is that this volume has stimulated the reader's imagination. Even more, we would be pleased if the discussions have contributed to a better understanding of the potential of a broad range of approaches to working with battered women and their families. The most satisfying result would be if the book helps to stimulate innovations and improvements in our approaches to helping.

References

Achenbach, T. M., & Edelbrock, C. S. (1983). *Manual for the child behavior checklist and revised child behavior profile.* Burlington, VT: Department of Psychiatry, University of Vermont.

Adam, B. D. (1978). *The survival of domination: Inferiorization and everyday life.* New York: Elsevier.

Adams, D. (1981). Counseling. In *Organizing and implementing services for men who batter* (pp. 19–46). Boston: Emerge, A Men's Counseling Service on Domestic Violence.

Adams, D. (1988). Treatment models of men who batter: A profeminist analysis. In M. Bograd & K. Yllo (Eds.), *Feminist perspectives on wife abuse* (pp. 176–199). Beverly Hills, CA: Sage.

Agle, L. E., & Pincus, L. D. (1977). A casework approach to police intervention in family disputes. *Social Casework, 58,* 43–45.

Aguirre, B. E. (1985, July–August). Why do they return? Abused wives in shelters. *Social Work,* 350–354.

Alinsky, S. D. (1971). *Rules for radicals.* New York: Vintage Books.

Allison, G. T. (1971). *Essence of decision: Explaining the Cuban missile crisis.* Boston: Little, Brown.

Atkeson, B. M., Forehand, R, & Rickard, K. M. (1982). The effects of divorce on children. In B. Lahey & A. E. Kazdin (Eds.), *Advances in clinical child psychology* (Vol. 5, pp. 255–281). New York: Plenum.

Avis, J. M. (1985). The politics of functional family therapy. Feminist Critique. *Journal of Marital and Family Therapy, 11*(2), 127–138.

Avis, J. M. (1988). Deepening awareness: A private study guide to feminism and family therapy. *Journal of Psychotherapy and the Family, 3,* 15–46.

Bagarozzi, D. A., & Giddings, W. C. (1983). Conjugal violence: A critical review of current research and clinical practices. *The American Journal of Family Therapy, 11*(1), 3–15.

Ball, P. G., & Wyman, E. (1977–1978). Battered wives and powerlessness: What can counselors do? *Victimology: An International Journal, 2,* 545–552.

Bandura, A. (1973). *Aggression: A social learning analysis.* Englewood Cliffs, NJ: Prentice-Hall.

Bandura, A. (1977). *Social learning theory.* Englewood Cliffs, NJ: Prentice-Hall.

Bard, M. (1969). Family intervention police teams as a community mental health resource. *The Journal of Criminal Law, Criminology and Police Science, 60,* 247–50.

Bard, M., & Zacker, J. (1971). The prevention of family violence: Dilemmas of community intervention. *Journal of Marriage and the Family, 33,* 677–682.

Bardwick, J. M., & Douvan, E. (1972). Ambivalence: The socialization of women. In V. G. Gornick & B. K. Moran (Eds.), *Woman in sexist society: Studies in power and powerlessness* (pp. 225–241). New York: New American Library.

Barnsely, J., Jacobson, H. E., McIntosh, J., & Wintemute, M. J. (1980). *Review of Munroe house: Second stage housing for battered women.* Vancouver: Women's Research Centre.

Bass, D., & Rice, J. (1979, June). Agency responses to the abused wife. *Social Casework: The Journal of Contemporary Social Work, 60,* 338–342.

Beaudry, M. (1985). *Battered women.* Montreal: Black Rose Books.

Belsky, J. (1980). Child maltreatment: An ecological integration. *American Psychologist, 35*(4), 320–335.

Benjamin, D. A., & Adler, S. (1980). Wife abuse: Implications for socio-legal policy and practice. *Canadian Journal of Family Law, 3,* 339–367.

Berk, R. A., & Newton, P. J. (1985, April). Does arrest really deter wife battery? An effort to replicate the findings of the Minneapolis spouse abuse experiment. *American Sociological Review, 50,* 253–262.

Berk, R. A., Newton, P. J., & Berk, S. F. (1986). What a difference a day makes; An empirical study of the impact of shelters for battered women. *Journal of Marriage and the Family, 48,* 481–490.

Berk, S. F., & Loseke, D. R. (1980–1981). "Handling" family violence: Situational determinants of police arrest in domestic disturbances. *Law and Society Review, 15,* 317–346.

Berkeley Planning Associates. (1977). *Evaluation: National Demonstration Program in Child Abuse & Neglect.* Berkeley, CA: Author.

Bloom, M. (1981). *Primary prevention: The possible science.* Englewood Cliffs, NJ: Prentice-Hall.

Bograd, M. (1984). Family systems approaches to wife battering: A feminist critique. *American Journal of Orthopsychiatry, 54,* 558–568.

Borkin, J., & Siegel, S. (1983). Primary prevention: Issues in curriculum development. In J.P. Bowker (Ed.), *Education for primary prevention in social work* (pp. 24–37). New York: Council on Social Work Education.

Borkowski, M., Murch, M., & Walker, V. (1983). *Marital violence: The community response.* London: Tavistock.

Bowen, M. (1978). *Family therapy in clinical practice.* New York: Jason Aronson.

Bowker, J.P. (Ed.) (1983). *Education for primary prevention in social work.* New York: Council on Social Work Education.

Bowker, L. H. (1982). Police services to battered women. *Criminal Justice and Behaviour, 9,* 476–494.

Bowker, L.H. (1983). *Beating wife-beating.* Toronto: Lexington.

Bowker, L.H. (1986). *Ending the violence.* Holmes Beach, FL: Learning Publications.

Bowker, L. H., & Maurer, L. (1985). The importance of sheltering in the lives of battered women. *Response, 8,* 2–8.

Bowker, L. H., & Maurer, L. (1987). The medical treatment of battered wives. *Women and Health, 12*(1), 25–45.

Bream, L., Hymel, S., & Rubin, K. (1986). *The social information problem solving interview: A manual for administration and scoring.* Unpublished manuscript, University of Waterloo, Department of Psychology, Waterloo, Ontario.

Breines, W., & Gordon, L. (1983). The new scholarship on family violence. *Journal of Women in Culture and Society, 8*(3) 492–531.

Brennan, A. F. (1985). Political and psychosocial issues in psychotherapy for spouse abusers: Implications for treatment. *Psychotherapy, 22,* 643–654.

Brody, C. M. (Ed.). (1984). *Women therapists working with women: New theory and process of feminist therapy.* New York: Springer.

Broemling, R. (1986). Family consultant service with the London police force. *The Reporter* (Ontario Social Development Council), *31,* 14.

Bronfenbrenner, U. (1979). *The ecology of human development.* Cambridge, MA : Harvard University Press.

Brown, R. (1986). *Social psychology: The second edition.* New York: The Free Press.

Browne, S. G. (1980). *In sickness and in health: Analysis of a battered women population.* Denver, CO: Denver Anti-Crime Council.

Brownell, A., & Shumaker, S. A. (1985). Where do we go from here? The policy implications of social support. *Journal of Social Issues, 41*(1), 111–121.

Browning, J. (1984). *Stopping the violence: Canadian programmes for assaultive men.* Ottawa: National Clearinghouse on Family Violence, Health and Welfare Canada.

Brownmiller, S. (1975). *Against our will: Men, women and rape.* Toronto: Bantam Books.

Burghardt, S. (1982). *The other side of organizing.* Cambridge, MA: Schenkonan Publishing.

Burris, C. A., & Jaffe, P. (1983). Wife abuse as a crime: The impact of police laying charges. *Canadian Journal of Criminology, 25,* 309–318.

Burris, C.A., & Jaffe, P. (1984). Wife battering: A well-kept secret. *Canadian Journal of Criminology, 26,* 171–177.

Byles, J. A. (1980). Family violence in Hamilton. *Canada's Mental Health, 28*(1), 4–6.

Byles, J. A. (1982). Family violence in Hamilton—Revisited. *Canada's Mental Health, 30*(4), 10–11.

Byles, J. A., Byrne, C., Boyle, M. H., & Offord, D. R. (1988). The General Functioning Scale of the Family Assessment Device: Reliability and validity. *Family Process, 27*, 97–104.

Cameron, G. (in press). The potential of informal social support strategies in child welfare. In M. Rothery & G. Cameron (Eds.), *Child maltreatment: Expanding our concept of helping.* Hillsdale, NJ: Lawrence Erlbaum Associates.

Cameron, G. (1985). Social action. In S. Yelaja (Ed.), *An introduction to social work practice in Canada* (pp. 111–133). Toronto: Prentice-Hall Canada.

Canada, House of Commons. (1986). *Debates,* May 16.

Canadian Council on Social Development (1982). *A reader on prevention and social policies.* Ottawa: CCSD.

Caplan, G. (1964). *Principles of preventive psychiatry.* New York: Basic.

Caplan, P. J. (1984). The myth of women's masochism. *American Psychologist, 39*(2), 130–139.

Caplan, P. J. (1987). *The myth of women's masochism.* New York: Signet.

Caplan, P. J., & Hall-McCorquodale, I. (1985). Mother-blaming in major clinical journals. *American Journal of Orthopsychiatry, 55*, 345–353.

Carlson, B. E. (1977, November). Battered women and their assailants. *Social Work, 22*, 445–465.

Carlson, B. E. (1984). Children's observations of interparental violence. In A. R. Roberts (Ed.), *Battered women and their families* (pp. 147–167). New York: Springer.

Chekki, D. A. (1979). *Community development.* New Delhi, India: Vikas Publishing House, P. V. T.

Chesler, P. (1973). *Women and madness.* New York: Avon.

Chodorow, N. (1978). *The reproduction of mothering.* Berkeley: University of California Press.

Christopoulos, C., Cohn, D., Sullivan-Hanson, J., Kraft, S. P., & Emery, R. E. (1985, April). *School-aged children's psychological adjustment to spouse abuse.* Paper presented at the meeting of the Society for Research in Child Development, Toronto, Canada.

Claerhout, S., Elder, J., & Janes, C. (1982). Problem-solving skills of rural battered women. *American Journal of Community Psychology, 10*, 605–613.

Cloward, R., & Piven, F. F. (1977). The acquiescence of social work. *Society, 14*(2), 55–62.

Cohen, S., & Wills, T. A. (1985). Stress, social support, and the buffering hypothesis. *Psychological Bulletin, 98*(2), 310–357.

Colbach, E. M., & Fosterling, C. D. (1976). *Police social work.* Springfield, IL: Charles C. Thomas.

Coleman, K. W. (1980). Conjugal violence: What 33 men report. *Journal of Marital and Family Therapy, 6*, 207–213.

Colorado Association for Aid to Battered Women. (1978). *Monograph on services to battered women.* Washington, DC: Department of HEW Office of Domestic Violence.

Conn, J. H., & Kanner, L. (1947). Children's awareness of sex differences. *Journal of Child Psychiatry, 1,* 3–57.

Cook, D. R., & Frantz-Cook, A. (1984). A systemic treatment approach to wifebattering. *Journal of Marital and Family Therapy, 10*(1), 83–93.

Craft, J., & Wynn, M. (1985). *Second stage housing: Assessing the need in Saint John* (research project). New Brunswick: Canada Employment and Immigration Commission and Department of Social Services.

Cummings, E. M., Iannotti, R. J., & Zahn-Waxler, C. (1985). Influence of conflict between adults on the emotions and aggression of young children. *Developmental Psychology, 21,* 495-507.

Daly, M. (1978). *Gyn/Ecology: The metaethics of radical feminism.* Boston: Beacon Press.

Davidson, T. (1977). Wifebeating: A recurring phenomenon throughout history. In M. Roy (Ed.), *Battered women: A psychosociological study of domestic violence* (pp. 2–23). New York: Van Nostrand Reinhold.

Davidson, T. (1978). *Conjugal crime understanding and changing the wifebeating pattern.* New York: Ballantine Books.

Deutsch, H. (1944). *The psychology of women* (Vol. 1). New York: Grune & Stratton.

Dobash, R. E., & Dobash R. P. (1977–1978). Wives: The 'appropriate' victims of marital violence. *Victimology: An International Journal, 2,* 426–442.

Dobash, R. E., & Dobash, R. P. (1979). *Violence against wives: A case against the patriarchy.* New York: The Free Press.

Dobash, R. E., Dobash, R. P., & Cavanaugh, K. (1985). The contact between battered women and social and medical agencies. In J. Pahl (Ed.), *Private violence and public policy. The needs of battered women and the response of the public services* (pp. 142–165). Boston: Routledge & Kegan Paul.

Dodge, K. A. (1986). A social information processing model of social competence in children. In M. Perlmutter (Ed.), *Minnesota Symposium on Child Psychology* (Vol. 18, pp. 77–125). Hillsdale, NJ: Lawrence Erlbaum Associates.

Dolan, R., Hendricks, J., & Meagher, S. (1986). Police practices and attitudes toward domestic violence. *Journal of Police Science and Administration, 14*(3), 187–192.

Doyle, J. A. (1983). *The male experience.* Dubuque, IA: Wm. C. Brown.

Dutton, D. G. (1987). The criminal justice response to wife assault. *Law and Human Behavior, 11*(3), 189–206.

Dutton, D. G., & Painter, S. L. (1981). Traumatic bonding: The development of emotional attachments in battered women and other relationships of intermittent abuse. *Victimology: An International Journal, 6*(1–4), 139–155.

Dutton, D.G. (1983). A nested ecological theory of male violence towards intimates. In P. Caplan (Ed.), *Feminist psychology in transition* (pp. 43–65). Montreal: Eden Press.

Dutton, D. G. (1984a). *The criminal justice system response to wife assault.* Ottawa: Ministry of the Solicitor General of Canada.

Dutton, D. G. (1984b). Interventions into the problem of wife assault: Therapeutic, policy and research implications. *Canadian Journal of Behavioral Science, 16*(4), 281–297.

Dutton, D. G., & Browning, J. (1983). Violence in intimate relationships. *International society for research on aggression,* Victoria, British Columbia.

Eddy, M. J., & Myers, T. (1984). *Helping men who batter: Profile of programs in the U. S.* Paper presented at the Second Conference on Family Violence, Durham, NH.

Edleson, J., & Grusznski, R. (1986). Treating men who batter: Four years of outcome data from the Domestic Abuse Project. Minneapolis: MI: Domestic Abuse Project, unpublished report.

Edmunson, E. D., Bedel, J. R., & Gordon, R. C. (1984). The community development project. In A. Gartner & F. Riessman (Eds.), *The self help revolution.* New York: Human Sciences Press.

Eekelaar, J. M., & Katz, S. N. (1978). *Family violence: An international and interdisciplinary study.* Toronto: Butterworth.

Eisenberg, S. E., & Micklow, P. L. (1976). *The assaulted wife: 'Catch 22' revisited.* Ann Arbor: University of Michigan Law School.

Elbow, M. (1982). Children of violent marriages: The forgotten victims. *Social Casework, 63,* 465–471.

Ellenberger, H. (1970). *The discovery of the unconscious: The history and evolution of dynamic psychiatry.* New York: Basic.

Ellis, J. (1984). Prosecutorial discretion to charge in cases of spousal assault: A dialogue. *The Journal of Criminal Law and Criminology, 75,* 56–102.

Eme, R. F. (1979). Sex differences in childhood psychopathology: A review. *Psychological Bulletin, 86,* 574–595.

EMERGE. (1981). *Organizing and implementing services for men who batter.* Boston: Author.

Emery, R. E., Kraft, S. P., Joyce, S., & Shaw, D. (1986, August). *Children of abused women: Adjustment at four months following shelter residence.* Paper presented at the meeting of the American Psychological Association, Washington, DC.

Eron, L. D. (1987). The development of aggressive behavior from the perspective of a developing behaviorism. *American Psychologist, 42,* 435–442.

Fagan, J. A., Stewart, D. A., & Hansen, K. V. (1983). Violent men or violent husbands? Background factors and situational correlates. In D. Finkelhor, R. J Gelles, G. T. Hotaling, & M. A. Straus (Eds.), *The dark side of families: Current family violence research* (pp. 49–67). Beverly Hills: Sage.

Faulk, M. (1974). Men who assault their wives. *Medicine, Science and the Law, 7*(2), 180–183.

Feazell, C., Mayers, R., & Deschner, J. (1984, April). Services for men who batter: implications for programs and policies. *Family Relations, 33,* 217–223.

Ferraro, K. J. (1981). Processing battered women. *Journal of Family Issues, 2*(4), 415–438.

Ferraro, K. J., & Johnson, J. M. (1983). How women experience battering: The process of victimization. *Social Problems, 30*(3), 325–339.

Field, M. H., & Field, H. F. (1973). Marital violence and the criminal process: Neither justice nor peace. *Social Service Review, 47*, 221–240.

Finkelhor, D. (1983). Common features of family abuse. In D. Finkelhor, R. J. Gelles, G. T. Hotaling, & M. A. Straus (Eds.), *The dark side of families: Current family violence research* (pp. 17–30). Beverly Hills: Sage.

Finkelhor, D. (1984). *Child sexual abuse: New theory and research*. New York: The Free Press.

Fleming, J. (1979). *Stopping wife abuse*. New York: Anchor Books.

Flynn, J. P. (1977, January). Recent findings related to wife abuse. *Social Casework, 58*, 13–20.

Ford, D. A. (1983, October). Wife battery and criminal justice: A study of victim decision-making. *Family Relations, 32*, 463–475.

Framo, J. L. (1976). Family of origin as a therapeutic resource for adults in family and marital therapy: You can and should go home again. *Family Process, 15*, 193–210.

Freeman, M. D. A. (1979). *Violence in the home*. Farnborough: Saxon House.

Freeman, M. D. A. (1977). Le vice anglais? Wife battering in English and American law. *Family Law Quarterly, 11*, 199–251.

Freeman, M. D. A. (1980). Violence against women: Does the legal system provide solutions or itself constitute the problem? *Canadian Journal of Family Law, 3*, 377–401.

Freud, S. (1959). Some psychological consequences of the anatomical distinction between the sexes. In J. Strachey (Ed.), *The collected papers of Sigmund Freud* (Vol. 5, pp. 186–197). New York: Basic.

Freud, S. (1965). Femininity. In J. Strachey (Ed.), *The new introductory lectures on psychoanalysis* (pp. 81–111). New York: Norton.

Friedrich, W. N., & Boriskin, J. A. (1982). The role of the child in abuse: A review of the literature. In G. J. Williams & J. Money (Eds.), *Traumatic abuse and neglect of children at home* (abridged ed. pp. 160–171). Baltimore MD: Johns Hopkins University Press.

Friere, P. (1981). *Pedagogy of the oppressed*. New York: Continuum.

Frieze, I. H., Knoble, J., Washburn, & Zomnir, G. (1980). *Characteristics of battered women and their marriages*. Pittsburgh, PA: University of Pittsburgh, Department of Psychology.

Froland, C., Pancoast, D., Chapman, N., & Kimboko, P. (1981). *Helping networks and human services*. Beverly Hills, CA: Sage.

Ganley, A.L. (1981). *Court-mandated counseling for men who batter: A three-day workshop for mental health professionals*. Washington, DC: Center for Women Policy Studies.

Garbarino, J. (1977). The human ecology of child maltreatment. *Journal of Marriage and the Family, 39*(6), 721–735.

Garbarino, J., & Gilliam, G. (1980). *Understanding abusive families*. Lexington, MA: Lexington Books.

Garmezy, N. (1983). Stressors of Childhood. In N. Garmezy & M. Rutter (Eds.), *Stress, Coping, & Development in Children* (pp. 43–84). New York: McGraw-Hill.

Garner, G. W. (1979). *The police role in alcohol-related crises*. Springfield, IL: Charles C. Thomas.

Gayford, J. J. (1975). Battered wives. *Medicine, Science and the Law, 15,* 288–289.

Geismar, L.C. (1969). *Preventive intervention in social work.* Metuchen, NJ: The Scarecrow Press.

Gelinas, D. J. (1983). The persisting negative effects of incest. *Psychiatry, 46,* 312–332.

Geller, J. A. (1978). Reaching the battering husband. *Social Work with Groups, 1,* 27–37.

Geller, J. A., & Wasserstrom, J. (1984). Conjoint therapy for the treatment of domestic violence. In A. R. Roberts (Ed.), *Battered women and their families* (pp. 33–48). New York: Springer.

Gelles, R. J. (1974). *The violent home.* Beverly Hills, CA: Sage.

Gelles, R. (1976). Abused wives: Why do they stay? *Journal of Marriage and the Family, 38*(4), 659–668.

Gelles, R. J., & Cornell, C. P. (1983). *International perspectives on family violence.* Lexington, MA: D. C. Heath.

Gelles, R. J., & Cornell, C. P. (1985). *Intimate violence in families. Family studies text series* (Vol. 2). Beverly Hills, CA: Sage.

Gelles, R. J., & Straus, M. A. (1979). Determinants of violence in the family: Toward a theoretical integration. In W. Burr, R. Mill, F. I. Nye, & I.L. Reiss (Eds.), *Contemporary theories about the family (549–581).* New York: The Free Press.

George, V., & Wilding, P. (1985). *Ideology and social welfare.* London: Routledge & Kegan Paul.

Giarretto, H. (1976). Humanistic treatment of father–daughter incest. In R. E. Helfer & C. H. Kempe (Eds.), *Child abuse and neglect: The family and the community* (pp. 15–28). Cambridge, MA: Ballinger.

Giarretto, H. (1982). A comprehensive child sexual abuse treatment program. *Child Abuse and Neglect, 6,* 263–278.

Gil, D. (1986). Sociocultural aspects of domestic violence. In M. Lystad (Ed.), *Violence in the home: Interdisciplinary perspectives* (pp. 124–149). New York: Brunner/Mazel.

Giles-Sims, J. (1983). *Wife battering: A systems theory approach.* New York: Guilford Press.

Giles-Sims, J. (1985). A longitudinal study of battered children of battered wives. *Family Relations, 34*(2), 205–219.

Gilligan, C. (1982). *In a different voice.* Cambridge, MA: Harvard University Press.

Gitterman, A., & Germain, C.B. (1976). Social work practice: A life model. *Social Service Review, 50*(4), 601–610.

Goldberg, D. P., & Hillier, V. F. (1979). A scaled version of the General Health Questionnaire. *Psychological Medicine, 9,* 139–145.

Goldner, V. (1985a). Feminism and family therapy. *Family Process, 24,* 31–47.

Goldner, V. (1985b). Warning: Family therapy may be hazardous to your health. *The Family Therapy Networker, 9,* 19–23.

Goldstein, A. P., Monti, P. J., Sardmo, T. J., & Green, D. J. (1977). *Police crisis intervention.* Kalamazoo, MI: Behaviordelia.

Gondolf, E. W. (1985a). *Men who batter: An integrated approach for stopping wife abuse.* Holmes Beach, FL: Learning Publications.

Gondolf, E. W. (1985b). Anger and oppression in men who batter: Empiricist and feminist perspectives and their implications for research. *Victimology: An International Journal, 10*(1–4), 311–324.

Gondolf, E. W. (1985c). Fighting for control: A clinical assessment of men who batter. *Social Casework: The Journal of Contemporary Social Work, 66,* 48–54.

Gondolf, E. W. (1987). Evaluating programs for men who batter: Problems and prospects. *Journal of Family Violence, 2*(1), 95–108.

Gondolf, E. W., & Hanneken, J. (1987). The gender warrior: Reformed batterers on abuse, treatment, and change. *Journal of Family Violence, 2*(2), 177–191.

Gondolf, E. W., & Russell, D. (1986). The case against anger control treatment programs for batterers. *Response, 9,* 2–5.

Goode, W. (1971, November). Force and violence in the family. *Journal of Marriage and the Family, 33,* 624–636.

Greenspan, M. (1983). *A new approach to women and therapy.* Toronto: McGraw-Hill.

Groth, A. N. (1982) The incest offender. In S. M. Sgroi (Ed.), *Handbook of clinical intervention in child sexual abuse* (pp. 215–239). Lexington, MA: Lexington Books.

Grunebaum, H., & Belfer, M. (1986). What family therapists might learn from child psychiatry. *Journal of Marital and Family Therapy, 12,* 415–423.

Hammen, C., Adrian, C., Gordon, D., Burge, D., Jaenicke, C., & Hiroto, D. (1987). Children of depressed mothers: Maternal strain and symptom predictors of dysfunction. *Journal of Abnormal Psychology, 96,* 190–198.

Hanks, S. E., & Rosenbaum, C. P. (1977). Battered women: A study of women who live with violent alcohol-abusing men. *American Journal of Orthopsychiatry, 47,* 291–306.

Hare-Mustin, R. T. (1978). A feminist approach to family therapy. *Family Process, 17,* 181–193.

Head, W. A. (1979). Community development in post-industrial society: Myth or reality. In D. A. Chekki (Ed.), *Community development* (pp. 101–113). New Delhi, India: Vikas Publishing House.

Health and Welfare Canada. (1986). *Canadian treatment programmes for men who batter.* Ottawa: National Clearinghouse on Family Violence.

Health and Welfare Canada. (1987). *Transition houses and shelters for battered women in canada.* Ottawa: National Clearinghouse on Family Violence.

Hendricks, D. R., & Meagher, M. S. (1986). Police Practices and attitudes towards domestic violence. *Journal of Police Science and Administration, 14*(3), pp. 187–192.

Hershorn, M., & Rosenbaum, A. (1985). Children of marital violence: A closer look at the unintended victims. *American Journal of Orthopsychiatry, 55,* 260–266.

Hess, R. D., & Camera, K. A. (1979). Post-divorce family relations as mediating factors in the consequences of divorce for children. *Journal of Social Issues, 35,* 79-98.

Hetherington, E. M., Cox, M., & Cox, R. (1979). Family interaction and the social, emotional and cognitive development of children following divorce. In V. Vaughn & T. Brazelton (Eds.), *The family: Setting priorities* (pp. 105–121). New York: Science & Medicine.

Hetherington, E. M., Cox, M., & Cox, R. (1982). Effects of divorce on parents and children. In M. E. Lamb (Ed.), *Nontraditional families: Parenting and child development* (pp. 233–288). Hillsdale, NJ: Lawrence Erlbaum Associates.

Hill, M. H., & Jackson, D. N. (1984). Parallel forms for the Basic Personality Inventory. *Research Bulletin, 616,* Dept. of Psychology, University of Western Ontario.

Hofeller, K. H. (1982). *Social, psychological, and situational factors in wife abuse.* Palo Alto, CA: R & E Research Associates.

Hoffman, L. (1981). *Foundations of family therapy: A conceptual framework for systems change.* New York: Basic Books.

Holmes, S. A. (1982). A Detroit model for police-social work cooperation. *Social Casework, 63,* 220–236.

Hughes, H. M., & Barad, S. J. (1982). Changes in the psychological functioning of children in a battered women's shelter: A pilot study. *Victimology,* 4(1-4), 60-68.

Hughes, H. M., & Barad, S. J. (1983). Psychological functioning of children in a battered women's shelter: A preliminary investigation. *American Journal of Orthopsychiatry, 53,* 525-531.

Hughes, J. M., & Hampton, K. L. (1984). *Relationships between the affective functioning of physically abused and nonabused children and their mothers in shelters for battered women.* Paper presented at the 92nd Annual Convention of the American Psychological Association, Toronto, Canada.

Jaffe, P., & Burris, C. A. (1982). *An integrated response to wife assault: A community model.* Ottawa: Ministry of the Solicitor General of Canada.

Jaffe, P., Finlay, T. J., & Wolfe, D. A. (1984). Evaluating the impact of a specialized civilian family crisis unit within a police force on the resolution of family conflicts. *Journal of Preventive Psychiatry, 2,* 63–73.

Jaffe, P., Wilson, S., & Wolfe, D. A. (1986). Promoting changes in attitudes and understanding of conflict resolution among child witnesses of family violence. *Canadian Journal of Behavioral Science, 18,* 356–365.

Jaffe, P., Wolfe, D. A., Telford, A., & Austin, G. (1986). The impact of police charges in incidents of wife abuse. *Journal of Family Violence, 1,* 37–49.

Jaffe, P., Wolfe, D. A., Wilson, S.K., & Zak, L. (1985). Critical issues in the assessment of children's adjustment to witnessing family violence. *Canada's Mental Health, 33*(4), 15-19.

Jaffe, P., Wolfe, D. A., Wilson, S. K. & Zak, L. (1986a). Family violence and child adjustment: A comparative analysis of girl's and boy's behavioral symptoms. *American Journal of Psychiatry, 143,* 74-77.

Jaffe, P., Wolfe, D. A., Wilson, S. K., & Zak, L. (1986b). Similarities in behavioral and social maladjustment among child victims and witnesses to family violence, *American Journal of Orthopsychiatry, 56,* 142–146.

Jaggar, A.M. (1983). *Feminist politics and human nature.* Totowa, NJ: Rowan & Allanheld.

James, K., & McIntyre, D. (1983). The reproduction of families: The social role of family therapy? *Journal of Marital and Family Therapy, 9,* 119–129.

Jennings, J. L. (1987). History and issues in the treatment of battering men: A case for unstructured group therapy. *Journal of Family Violence, 3,* 193–213.

Johnson, K. W. (1977). *Police interagency relations: Some research findings.* Beverly Hills: Sage.

Johnson, J. M. (1981). Program enterprise and official cooptation in the battered women's shelter movement. *American Behavioral Scientist,* 24(6), 827–842.

Jouriles, E. N., Barling, J., & O'Leary, K. D. (1987). Predicting child behavior problems in maritally violent families. *Journal of Abnormal Child Psychology, 15,* 165–173.

Katcher, A. (1955). The discrimination of sex differences by young children. *Journal of Genetic Psychology, 85,* 131–143.

Katz, S. (1986, November). How London, Ontario is calling a halt to wife abuse. *Chatelaine,* pp. 56 & 128.

Kaufman, J., & Zigler, E. (1987). Do abused children become abusive parents? *American Journal of Orthopsychiatry, 57,* 186–192.

Kendall, S. (1985). *Children in domestic violence: Final report.* Prepared for Win House, Edmonton, Women's Shelter.

Kennedy, D. B., & Homant, R. J. (1984). Battered women's evaluation of the police response. *Victimology: An International Journal, 9,* 174–79.

Kincaid, P. J. (1982). *The omitted reality: Husband-wife violence in Ontario and policy implications for education.* Concord, Ontario: Belsten Publishing.

Kleckner, J. (1978). Wife beaters and beaten wives: Co-conspirators in crimes of violence. *Psychology, 15,* 54–56.

Knowles, M. (1980). *Couple violence.* Kingston, Ontario: Frontenac Family Referral Service.

Knowles, M., & Middleton, B. (1980). *Violent couples.* Kingston, Ontario: Frontenac Family Referral Service.

Kuhl, A. F. (1982). Community responses to battered women. *Victimology: An International Journal, 7*(1–4), 49–59.

Langley, R., & Levy, R. C. (1977). *Wife beating: The silent crisis.* New York: E. P. Dutton.

LaPrairie, C. (1983). *Family violence in rural, northern communities: A proposal for research and program development.* Prepared for the Research Division, Programs Branch, Solicitor General Canada, Ottawa.

Leger, G. J. (1983). Family violence and the criminal justice system. *R. C. M. P. Gazette, 45,* 13–15.

Leger, G. J. (1984). *The criminal charges as a means of assisting victims of wife assault.* Ottawa: Ministry of the Solicitor General of Canada.

Lemmon, J. A. (1985). *Family mediation practice.* New York: The Free Press.

Lerette, P. (1984). *Study of the Restigouche family crisis interveners program.* Ottawa: Ministry of the Solicitor General of Canada.

Levens, B. R. (1978). *The social service role of police domestic crisis intervention.* Vancouver, B. C. : United Way of the Lower Mainland.

Levens, R. R., & Dutton, D. G. (1980). *The social service role of the police: Domestic crisis intervention.* Ottawa: Solicitor General of Canada.

Libow, J., Raskin, P., & Caust, B. (1982). Feminism and family systems therapy: are they irreconcilable? *American Journal of Family Therapy, 10,* 3–12.

Lieber, L. L., & Baker, J. M. (1977). Parents Anonymous—Self-help treatment for child abusing parents: A review and an evaluation. *Child Abuse and Neglect, 1,* 133–148.

Lieberknecht, K. (1978, April). Helping the battered wife. *American Journal of Nursing,* 654–656.

Lion, J. (1977). Clinical aspects of wifebeating. In M. Roy (Ed.), *Battered women* (pp. 126–136). New York: Van Nostrand Reinhold.

London Battered Women's Advocacy Clinic Inc. (1985). *Final report,* London, Ontario: Author.

London Police Force. (1986). *1986 Annual report.* London: Author.

Long, N., & Forehand, R. (1987). The effects of parental divorce and parental conflict on children: An overview. *Developmental and Behavioral Pediatrics, 8,* 292–297.

Lorion, R.P. (1983). Research issues in the design and evaluation of preventive interventions. In J.P. Bowker (Ed.), *Education for primary prevention in social work* (pp. 7–23). New York: Council on Social Work Education.

Loseke, D. R., & Cahill, S. R. (1984). The social construction of deviance: Experts on battered women. *Social Problems, 31*(3), 296–310.

Loseke, D. R., & Berk, S. F. (1982). The work of shelters; Battered women and initial calls for help. *Victimology: An International Journal, 7,* 35–48.

Loving, N. (1980). *Responding to spouse abuse and wife beating: A guide for police.* Washington, DC: Police Executive Research Forum.

Loving, N. (1981). *Spouse abuse: A curriculum guide for police trainers.* Washington, DC: Police Research Forum.

Lystad, M. (1982). Violence in the home: A major public problem. *Urban and Social Change Review, 3,* 21–25.

Lystad, M. (Ed.). (1986). *Violence in the home: Interdisciplinary perspectives.* New York: Brunner/Mazel.

MacKinnon, L. K., & Miller, D. (1987). The new epistemology and the Milan approach: Feminist and sociopolitical considerations. *Journal of Marital and Family Therapy, 13*(2), 139–155.

MacLeod, L. (1979). *Task force on family violence.* Vancouver. Vancouver Social Planning and Research.

MacLeod, L. (1980). *Wife battering in Canada: The vicious cycle.* Ottawa: Canadian Advisory Council on the Status of Women.

MacLeod, L. (1986). *Transition house: How to establish a refuge for battered women.* Ottawa: Health & Welfare Canada.

MacLeod, L. (1987). *Battered but not beaten: Preventing wife battering in Canada.* Ottawa: Canadian Advisory Council on the Status of Women.

Magill, J., & Werk, A. (1985). A treatment model for marital violence. *The Social Worker, 53*(2), 61–64.

Maidment, S. (1980). The relevance of the criminal law to domestic violence. *Journal of Social Welfare Law,* 26–32.

Margolin, G. (1979). Conjoint marital therapy to enhance anger management and reduce spouse abuse. *American Journal of Family Therapy, 7,* 13–23.

Martin, D. (1976). *Battered wives.* San Francisco: Blide Publications.

Martin, D. (1978). Battered women: society's problem. In J. R. Chapman & M. Gates (Eds.), *The victimization of women* (pp. 111–141). Beverley Hills, CA: Sage.

Masson, J. M. (1985). *The assault on truth.* New York: Penguin.

Masters, W. H., & Johnson, V. E. (1966). *Human sexual response.* Boston: Little, Brown.

McCafferty, M. (1983). *Making connections: Feminist therapy and social work.* Unpublished masters research project, Faculty of Social Work, Wilfrid Laurier University, Waterloo, Ontario.

McCall, G. J., & Simmons, J. L. (1966). *Identities and interactions.* New York: The Free Press.

McCormick, A. J. (1981). A review of literature and Emerge's view of the problem. In *Organizing and implementing services for men who batter* (pp. 1–13). Boston: EMERGE, A men's counseling service on domestic violence.

McDonald, L., Chisholm, W., Peressini, T., & Smillie, T. (1986). *A review of a second stage shelter for battered women and their children.* Funded by the National Welfare Grants Directorate, Health and Welfare Canada Project #4558–32–2.

McFall, R. M. (1982). A review and reformulation of the concept of social skills. *Behavioral Assessment, 4,* 1–33.

McKnight, J. (1977). Professionalized service and disabling help. In I. Illich, J. Mcknight, I. K. Zola, J. Caplan, & H. Shaiken (Eds.), *Disabling professions* (pp. 69–91). Great Britain: Marian Press.

McLaughlin, A. (1983). *An analysis of victims/victim-witness needs in Yukon.* Prepared for the Department of Justice Canada and the Department of Justice, Government of Yukon.

Meade-Ramrattan, J., Cerre, M. L., & Porto, M. L. (1980). Physically abused women: satisfaction with sources of help. *Social Worker, 48,* 162–166.

Miller, J. B. (1986). *Toward a new psychology of women* (2nd ed.). Boston: Beacon Press.

Milwaukee Task Force on Battered Women, Junior League of Milwaukee. (1982). *Domestic violence: The all-American crime: A collaborative model for community response.* Milwaukee: The League.

Minuchin, S. (1974). *Families and family therapy.* Cambridge, MA: Harvard University Press.

Minuchin, S. (1984). *Family kaleidoscope.* Cambridge, MA: Harvard University Press.

Minuchin, S., & Fishman, C. (1981). *Family therapy techniques.* Cambridge, MA: Harvard University Press.

Monahan, J. (Ed.). (1976). *Community mental health and the criminal justice system.* New York: Pergamon Press.

Moore, D. (Ed.). (1979). *Battered women.* Beverly Hills, CA: Sage.

Morash, M. (1986). Wife battering. *Criminal Justice Abstracts, 18,* 252–271.

Muir, J., & LeClaire, D. (1984). *A police response to domestic assaults.* Ottawa: Ministry of the Solicitor General of Canada.

Myers, C. (1984). *The family violence project: Some preliminary data on a treatment program for spouse abuse.* Paper presented at the Second Annual Conference on Research in Family Violence, Durham, NH.

Nadler, D. A., Hackman, R. J., & Lawler, E. E., III. (1979). *Managing organizational behaviour.* Boston: Little, Brown.

Nairne, K., & Smith, G. (1985). *Dealing with depression.* London, England: The Women's Press Ltd.

National Council of Welfare. (1979). *Women and poverty.* Ottawa: National Council of Welfare.

National Council of Welfare. (1988, April). *Poverty profile 1988.* Ottawa: Minister of Supply and Services Canada.

Neidig, P. H., & Friedman, D. H. (1984). *Spouse abuse: A treatment program for couples.* Champaign, IL: Research Press Company.

Nichols, M. P. (1987). *The self in the system: Expanding the limits of family therapy.* New York: Brunner/Mazel.

O'Brien, J. (1971, November). Violence in divorce prone families. *Journal of Marriage and the Family, 33,* 193–211.

Ontario, Ministry of Community and Social Services. (September 16, 1986). [Newsrelease: Scott and Sweeney announce major new initiatives to reduce family violence.] Toronto: Communications Group.

Pagelow, M. D. (1981). *Woman-battering: Victims and their experiences.* Beverly Hills, CA: Sage.

Pahl, J. (1979). Refuges for battered women: Social provision or social movement? *Journal of Voluntary Action Research, 8,* 25–35.

Pahl, J. (1982). Police response to battered women. *Journal of Social Welfare Law.* 337–43.

Pahl, J. (1985). *Private violence and public policy. The needs of battered women and the response of the public services.* Boston: Routledge & Kegan Paul.

Parkinson, G. C. (1980). Cooperation between police and social workers: Hidden issues. *Social Work, 25,* 12–18.

Penfold, P. S., & Walker, G. A. (1983). *Women and the psychiatric paradox.* Montreal: Eden Press.

Pepler, D., & Kates, M. (1987, June). *Educational interventions with children exposed to family violence.* Paper presented at the National Conference on Family Violence, St. Johns, New Brunswick.

Perry, D. G., Perry, L. C., & Rasmussen, P. (1986). Cognitive social learning mediators of aggression. *Child Development, 57,* 700–711.

Pizzey, E. (1974). *Scream quietly or the neighbors will hear.* Harmondsworth: Penguin.

Police family crisis intervention. (1983). Proceedings of a Conference: Family Consultant Service, London Police Force, Ontario Police College, Solicitor General of Canada, London, Ontario.

Police Foundation. (1977). *Domestic violence and the police, studies in Detroit and Kansas City*. Washington, DC: Author.

Porter, C. (1983). Blame, depression and coping in battered women. Vancouver, BC: University of British Columbia, Unpublished Doctoral Dissertation.

Pressman, B. (1984). *Family violence: Origins and treatment*. Guelph, Ontario: Office for Educational Practice, University of Guelph.

Pressman, B. (1987). The place of family of origin therapy in the treatment of wife abuse. In A. J. Hovestadt & M. Fine (Eds.), *Family of origin therapy: The family therapy collections*. (pp. 45–56). Rockville, MD: Aspen Publishers.

Pressman, B. (1989). Wife-abused couples: The need for comprehensive theoretical perspectives and integrated treatment models. *Journal of Feminist Family Therapy, 1*, 23-43.

Purdy, F., & Nickle, N. (1981). Practice principles for working with groups of men who batter. *Social Work with Groups, 4*, 111–112.

Rappaport, J. (1977). *Community psychology: Values, research and action*. New York: Holt, Rinehart & Winston.

Rawlings, E. I., & Carter, D. K. (Eds.). (1977). *Psychotherapy for women: Treatment toward equality*. Springfiled, IL: Charles C. Thomas.

Regina Women's Transition Society (1984). *Breaking silence: Descriptive report of a followup study of abused women using a shelter*. Regina, Saskatchewan: Author.

Report of the Royal Commission. (1970). *The status of women in Canada*. Ottawa: Information Canada.

Ridington, J. (1977–1978a). *Women in transition: A study of Vancouver transition house as an agent of change*. Unpublished master's thesis, University of British Columbia, Canada.

Ridington, J. (1977–1978b). The transition process: A feminist environment as reconstitutive milieu. *Victimology: An International Journal, 2*(3–4), 563–575.

Ridington, J. (1982). Providing services: The feminist way. In M. Fitzgerald, C. Guberman, & M. Wolfe (Eds.), *Still ain't satisfied, Canadian feminism today* (pp. 93–107). Toronto: Women's Press.

Roberts, A. R. (Ed.). (1984). *Battered women and their families: Intervention strategies and treatment programs* (Vol. 1). New York: Springer.

Roberts, A. R. (1984). Intervention with the abusive partner. In A. R. Roberts (Ed.), *Battered women and their families: Intervention strategies and treatment programs* (pp. 84–115). New York: Springer.

Roberts, A. R. (1987). Psychosocial characteristics of batterers: A study of 234 men charged with domestic violence offenses. *Journal of Family Violence, 2*(1), 81–93.

Roberts, H. (1979). *Community development: Learning and action*. Toronto: University of Toronto Press.

Rohrbaugh, J. B. (1979). *Women: Psychology's puzzle*. New York: Basic.

Rosenbaum, A., & O'Leary, K. D. (1981a). Children: The unintended victims of marital violence. *American Journal of Orthopsychiatry, 51*, 692–699.

Rosenbaum, A., & O'Leary, K. D. (1981b). Marital violence: Characteristics of abusive couples. *Journal of Consulting and Clinical Psychology, 49,* 63–71.

Rosenberg, M. S. (1984, August). *Intergenerational family violence: A critique and implications for witnessing children.* Paper presented at the Annual Convention of the American Psychological Association, Toronto, Canada.

Rosewater, L. B. (1982). *An MMPI profile for battered women.* Doctoral Dissertation for Union Graduate School, Ann Arbor, MI: Dissertation Abstracts.

Rothery, M. (in press). Family problems with multiproblem families. In M. Rothery & G. Cameron (Eds.), *Child Maltreatment: Expanding our concept of helping.* Hillsdale, NJ: Lawrence Erlbaum Associates.

Rothery, M., & Cameron, G. (1985). *Understanding family support in child welfare: A summary report.* Toronto: Ontario Ministry of Community and Social Services.

Rothery, M., & Cameron, G. (in press). *Child maltreatment: Expanding our concept of helping.* Hillsdale, NJ: Lawrence Erlbaum Associates.

Rounsaville, B. J. (1978). Theories in marital violence: Evidence from a study of battered women. *Victimology: An International Journal, 3*(1–2), 11–31.

Roy, M. (Ed.). (1977). *Battered women: A psychosociological study of domestic violence.* New York: Van Nostrand Reinhold.

Roy, M. (Ed.). (1982). *The abusive partner: An analysis of domestic battering.* New York: Van Nostrand Reinhold.

Roy, M. (1982). The psychosociology of abusive behavior. In M. Roy (Ed.), *The abusive partner: An analysis of domestic battering* (pp. 3–16). New York: Van Nostrand Reinhold.

Rutter, M. (1971). Parent–child separation: psychological effects on the children. *Journal of Child Psychology and Psychiatry, 12,* 233-260.

Rutter, M. (1983). Stress, coping, and development: Some issues and some questions. In N. Garmezy & M. Rutter (Eds.), *Stress, coping, and development in children* (pp. 1–41). New York: McGraw-Hill.

Rutter, M. (1987). Psychosocial resilience and protective mechanisms. *American Journal of Orthopsychiatry, 57,* 316–331.

Ryan, W. (1976). *Blaming the victim.* New York: Vintage Books.

Sample Survey and Data Bank Unit. (1984). *Breaking Silence: Descriptive Report of a Follow-Up Study of Abused Women Using a Shelter.* Regina, SA: University of Regina.

Saunders, D. G. (1984). Helping husbands who batter. *Social Casework, 65,* 347–353.

Saunders, D. G., & Hanusa, D. R. (1986). Cognitive-behavioral treatment of men who batter: The short-term effects of group therapy. *Journal of Family Violence, 1*(4), 357–372.

Schechter, S. (1982). *Women and male violence. The visions and struggles of the battered women's movement.* Boston: South End Press.

Schultz, L.G. (1960). The wife assaulter. *Corrective Psychiatry and Journal of Social Therapy, 6,* 103–111.

Schwartz, R. (1987). Our multiples selves. *The Family Therapy Networker, 11,* 24–31, 80–83.

Seligman, M.E.P. (1975). *Helplessness: On depression, development and death.* San Francisco: Freeman.

Shaevitz, M.H. (1984). *The superwoman syndrome.* New York: Warner.

Shainess, N. (1979). Vulnerability to violence: Masochism as a process. *American Journal of Psychotherapy, 33,* 174–189.

Shelters to receive extra $6 million. (1987, April 15). Kitchener-Waterloo Record, p. B-1.

Sherman, L. W., & Berk, R. A. (1984a). The specific deterrent effects of arrest for domestic assault. *American Sociological Review, 49*(2), 261–272.

Sherman, L. W., & Berk, R. A. (1984b). *The Minneapolis domestic violence experiment.* Washington, DC: Police Foundation Reports.

Shupe, A., Stacey, W. A., & Hazlewood, L. R. (1987). *Violent men, violent couples.* Toronto: D. C. Heath.

Siefert, K. (1983). Using concepts from epidemiology to teach prevention. In J.P. Bowker (Ed.), *Education for primary prevention in social work* (pp. 54–74). New York: Council on Social Work Education.

Sinclair, D. (1985). *Understanding wife assault: A training manual for counsellors and advocates.* Toronto: Government of Ontario.

Sines, J. O., Clarke, W. M., & Lauer, R. M. (1984). Home Environment Questionnaire. *Journal of Abnormal Child Psychology, 12,* 519–529.

Small, S. E. (1981). *The interactionist perspective on wife assault: A sociological 'rule of thumb'.* Paper presented at the Annual Meetings of the Sociology and Anthropology Association, Halifax, Nova Scotia.

Smith, D. E. (1975). An analysis of ideological structures and how women are excluded: Considerations for academic women. *Canadian Review of Sociology and Anthropology, 12,* 353–369.

Smith, M. D. (1985). *Woman abuse: The case for surveys by telephone* [The LaMarsh Research Programme Reports on Violence and Conflict Resolution, Report #12]. Toronto: York University.

Snell, J. E., Rosenwald, R. J., & Robey, A. (1964). The wifebeater's wife: A study of family interaction. *Archives of General Psychiatry, 2,* 107–112.

Snider, G., & Skoretz, A. (1983). *Social indicators as predictors for child maltreatment.* Unpublished masters research project, Faculty of Social Work, Wilfrid Laurier University, Waterloo, Ontario.

Snyder, D. K., & Fruchtman, L. A. (1981). Differential patterns of wife abuse; A data-based typology. *Journal of Consulting and Clinical Psychology, 49*(6), 878–885.

Snyder, D. K., & Scheer, N. S. (1981). Predicting disposition following brief residence at a shelter for battered women. *American Journal of Community Psychology, 9*(5), 559–566.

Sopp-Gilson, S. (1980). Children from violent homes. *Journal, Ontario Association of Children's Aid Societies, 23*(10), 1–5.

Stacey, W. A., & Shupe, A. (1984). *The family secret: domestic violence in America.* Boston: Beacon Press.

Standing Committee on Health, Welfare and Social Affairs. (1982). *Report on violence in the family: Wife battering.* Canada: House of Commons Canada.

Star, B. (1978). Comparing battered and non-battered women. *Victimology: An International Journal, 3*(1–2), 32–44.

Star, B. (1980). Patterns in family violence. *Social Casework, 61,* 339–346.

Star, B. (1983). *Helping the abuser: Intervening effectively in family violence.* New York: Family Service Association of America.

Stark, E., Flitcraft, A., & Frazier, W. (1979). Medicine and patriarchal violence: The social construction of a 'private' event. *International Journal of Health Services, 9,* 461–493.

Stark, R., & McEvoy, J. III. (1970). Middle class violence. *Psychology Today, 4*(11), 52–54, 110–112.

Statistics Canada. (1977). *Income distributions by size in Canada* (Catalogue 13–207, Annual, Table 70). Ottawa: Author.

Statistics Canada. (1982). *Homicide in Canada: A statistical synopsis.* Ottawa: Statistics Canada, Justice Statistics Division.

Statistics Canada, Labour Force Survey Division. (1985). [unpublished data cited in *Women in the labour force fact and fiction. Factsheet number 1.*] Toronto: Ontario Women's Directorate.

Steele, B. F., & Pollock, C. B. (1974). A psychiatric study of parents who abuse infants and small children. In R. E. Helfer & H. Kempe (Eds.), *The battered child* (pp. 89–133). Chicago: The University of Chicago Press.

Steinfeld, G. (1986). Spouse abuse: Clinical implications of research on the control of aggression. *Journal of Family Violence, 1*(2), 197-208.

Steinmetz, S. K. (1977). *Cycle of violence—assertive, aggressive, and abusive family interaction.* New York: Praeger.

Stone, L. H. (1984). Shelters for battered women: A temporary escape from danger or the first step toward divorce? *Victimology: An International Journal, 9*(2), 284–289.

Straus, M.A. (1973). A general systems theory approach to a theory of violence between family members. *Social Science Information, 12*(3), 105–125.

Straus, M. A. (1976). Sexual inequality, cultural norms, and wife beating. *Victimology: An International Journal, 1,* 54–76.

Straus, M.A. (1977). A sociological perspective on the prevention and treatment of wifebeating. In M. Roy (Ed.), *Battered women: A psychosociological study of domestic violence* (pp. 194–239). New York: Van Nostrand Reinhold.

Straus, M.A. (1977–1978). Wife beating: How common and why? *Victimology, 2,* 443–458.

Straus, M.A., Gelles, R.J., & Steinmetz, S.K. (1980). *Behind closed doors: Violence in the American family.* Garden City, NY: Anchor Books.

Studer, M. (1984). Wife beating as a social problem: The process of definition. *International Journal of Women's Studies, 7*(5), 412–422.

Sutton, J. (1978). The growth of the British movement for battered women. *Victimology: An International Journal, 2*(3–4), 576–584.

Taggart, M. (1985). The feminist critique in epistemological perspective: Questions of context in family therapy. *Journal of Marital and Family Therapy, 11*(2), 113–126.

Taub, N. (1983). Adult domestic violence: The law's response. *Victimology: An International Journal, 8*, 152–171.

Taylor, J. W. (1984). Structured conjoint therapy for spouse abuse cases. *Social Casework, 65*, 11–18.

Thomas, T. (1986). *The police and social workers.* Aldershot, Hants: Gower Publishing.

Thorman, G. (1980). *Family violence.* Springfield, IL: Charles C. Thomas.

Tierney, K. J. (1982). The battered women movement and the creation of the wife beating problem. *Social problems, 29*(3), 207–220.

Tomes, N. (1978). A "Torrent of abuse": Crimes of violence between working class men and women in London, 1840–1875. *Journal of Social History, 3*, 329–345.

Treger, H. (1975). *The police-social work team.* Springfield, IL: Charles C. Thomas.

Treger, H. (1981). Police-social work cooperation, problems and issues. *Social Casework, 62*, 426–433.

Trimble, D. (1986). Confronting responsibility: Men who batter their wives. In A. Gitterman & L. Shulman (Eds.), *Mutual aid groups and the life cycle* (pp. 229–243). Itasca, IL: F. E. Peacock.

Truninger, E. (1971). Marital violence: The legal solutions. *Hastings Law Journal, 23*, 259–276.

Turner, S. F., & Shapiro, C. H. (1986). Battered women: Mourning the death of a relationship. *Social Work, 31*, 372–376.

Urbain, E. S., & Kendall, P. C. (1980). Review of social-cognitive problem-solving interventions with children. *Psychological Bulletin, 88*, 109–143.

Ursel, E. J., & Farough, D. (1986). The legal and public response to the new wife abuse directive in Manitoba. *Canadian Journal of Criminology, 28*, 171–183.

Videka-Sherman, L. (1985, July 10). *Harriett M. Bartlett practice effectiveness project: Report to NASW board of directors.* Silver Springs, MD: National Association of Social Workers.

Vis-!-Vis. (1987, Winter). After the crisis. Follow-up programs for the survivors of family violence. *A National Newsletter on Family Violence*, pp. 1–9.

Wahler, R. G. (1983). Predictors of treatment outcome in parent training: Mother insularity and socioenconomic disadvantage. *Behavioral Assessment, 5*, 301–313.

Waites, E. A. (1977–1978). Female masochism and the enforced restriction of choice. *Victimology: An International Journal. 2*(3–4), 535–544.

Walker, L. E. (1977–1978). Battered women and learned helplessness. *Victimology: An International Journal, 2*, 525–534.

Walker, L. E. (1979). *The battered woman.* New York: Harper & Row.

Walker, L. E. (1983). The battered woman syndrome study. In D. Finkelhor, R. Gelles, G. Hotaling, & M. Straus (Eds.), *The dark side of families: Current family violence research* (pp. 31–48). Beverley Hills, CA: Sage.

Walker, L. E. (1984a). Battered women, psychology, and public policy. *American Psychologist, 39*(10), 1178–1182.

Walker, L. E. (1984b). *The battered woman syndrome.* New York: Springer.

Wallerstein, J. S., & Kelly, J. B. (1976). The effects of parental divorce: Experiences of the child in later latency. *American Journal of Orthopsychiatry, 46,* 256-269.

Wardell, L., Gillespie, D. L., & Lefler, A. (1983). Science and violence against wives. In D. Finkelhor, R. Gelles, G. Hotaling, & M. Straus (Eds.), *The dark side of families: Current family violence research* (pp. 69–84). Beverley Hills, CA: Sage.

Watzlawick, P., Beavin, J. H., & Jackson, D. D. (1967). *Pragmatics of human communication.* New York: Norton.

Watzlawick, P., Weakland, J., & Fisch, R. (1974). *Change: Principles of problem formation and problem resolution.* New York: Norton.

Weakland, J. (1983). Family therapy with individuals. *Journal of strategic and systemic therapies, 2,* 1–9.

Weisstein, N. (1972). Psychology constructs the female. In V. Gornick & B. K. Moran (Eds.), *Woman in sexist society* (pp. 207–224). New York: Mentor.

Weitzman, J., & Dreen, K. (1982, May). Wife beating: A view of the marital dyad. *Social Casework, 63*(5), 259–265.

Whittaker, J. (1983). Social support networks in child welfare. In J. Whittaker & J. Garbarino (Eds.), *Social support networks* (pp. 167–186). New York: Aldine.

Wilde-Stevens, M. (1985). *Preliminary report: Crisis line statistics.* Winnipeg: Prepared for the Manitoba Committee on Wife Abuse.

Wilden, A. (1972). *System and structure.* New York: Tavistock.

Wilensky, H. L., & Lebeaux, C.N. (1965). *Industrial society and social welfare.* New York: The Free Press.

Withorn, A. (1984). *Serving the people: Social services and social change.* New York: Columbia University Press.

Wolfe, D. A., Jaffe, P., Wilson, S. K., & Zak, L. (1985). Children of battered women: The relation of child behavior to family violence and maternal stress. *Journal of Consulting and Clinical Psychology, 53,* 657–665.

Wolfe, D. A., & Mosk, M. (1983). Behavioral comparisons of children from abusive and distressed families. *Journal of Clinical Psychology, 51,* 702–708.

Wolfe, D. A., Zak, L., Wilson, S. K., & Jaffe, P. (1986). Child witnesses to violence between parents: Critical issues in behavioral and social adjustment. *Journal of Abnormal Child Psychology, 14,* 95–104.

Women's Research Center. (1982). *A study of protection for battered women.* Vancouver: Author.

Wyckoff, H. (1977). *Solving women's problems.* New York: Grove.

Author Index

A

Achenbach, T. M., 77, 79
Adam, B. D., 159, 161, 163
Adams, D., 32, 38, 41, 44, 63, 134
Adler, S., 132
Adrian, C., 79
Aguirre, B. E., 93, 99, 102–103, 105, 122
Alinsky, S. D., 159
Allison, G. T., 157
Atkeson, B. M., 78
Austin, G., 128, 133, 152, 154
Avis, J. M., 16–17, 24, 43–44, 140, 144

B

Bagarozzi, D. A., 47, 49–51, 53–54
Baker, J. M., 163
Ball, P. G., 96
Bandura, A., 61
Barad, S. J., 76
Bardwick, J. M., 14–15
Barling, J., 76
Barnsely, J., 119–121
Bass, D., 104
Beaudry, M., 111–112, 114–116
Beavin, J. H., 36

Bedel, J. R., 163
Belfer, M., 37
Belsky, J., 143
Benjamin, D. A., 132
Berk, R. A., 98, 102, 104, 107, 118, 122, 128, 152, 154
Berk, S. F., 102, 118–119, 121–122, 127
Berkeley Planning Associates, 163
Bloom, M., 138–139
Bograd, M., 16–17, 36, 47–49, 54, 63, 144
Boriskin, J. A., 9
Borkin, J., 138
Bowen, M., 37
Bowker, L. H., 102, 104–105, 122, 127, 133
Boyle, M. H., 70
Bream, L., 82
Breines, W., 141
Brennan, A. F., 38–39, 41
Brody, C. M., 44
Broemling, R., 131
Bronfenbrenner, U., 159, 163
Brown, R., 159, 163
Browne, S. G., 93
Brownell, A., 63
Browning, J., 58, 62, 64, 100, 138–140
Brownmiller, S., 42
Burge, D., 79

Burghardt, S., 158
Burris, C. A., 18, 80, 104, 125–126, 152, 154
Byles, J. A., 58, 70, 140
Byrne, C., 70

C

Cahill, S. R., 94, 103, 105–106
Camera, K. A., 77
Cameron, G., 158–159, 163
Caplan, G., 138
Caplan, P. J., 13, 16, 23, 95
Carlson, B. E., 80, 95, 120
Carter, D. K., 42, 44
Caust, B., 144–145
Cavanaugh, K., 104
Cerre, M. L., 31
Chapman, N., 163
Chekki, D. A., 158
Chesler, P., 30–31
Chisholm, W., 93, 95–96, 98, 100, 102, 106–107, 114, 119, 120–122
Chodorow, N., 43
Christopoulos, C., 76, 85
Claerhout, S., 78
Clarke, W. M., 83
Cloward, R., 159
Cohen, S., 163
Cohn, D., 76, 85
Coleman, K. W., 23
Conn, J. H., 31
Cook, D. R., 38, 47–54
Cornell, C. P., 100, 105
Cox, M., 76–77
Cox, R., 76–77
Craft, J., 119
Cummings, E. M., 78

D

Daly, M., 142
Davidson, T., 32, 142
Deschner, J., 65, 69
Deutsch, H., 31

Dobash, R. E., 9, 21, 36, 42, 44, 93, 95–96, 102, 104, 113, 125, 127, 139, 142
Dobash, R. P., 9, 21, 36, 42, 44, 93, 95–96, 102, 104, 113, 125, 127, 139, 142
Dodge, K. A., 82
Dolan, R., 104
Douvan, E., 14–15
Doyle, J. A., 11
Dreen, K., 49–51, 53
Dutton, D. G., 96, 98–100, 104, 107, 125, 132, 139, 144

E

Edelbrock, C. S., 77, 79
Edleson, J., 69
Edmunson, E. D., 163
Eisenberg, S. E., 100
Elbow, M., 24
Elder, J., 78
Ellenberger, H., 3
Ellis, J., 132
Eme, R. F., 80
Emery, R. E., 76, 78, 85
Eron, L. D., 77

F

Fagan, J. A., 60
Farough, D., 104, 132
Faulk, M., 94–95
Feazell, C., 65, 69
Ferraro, K. J., 93, 96, 98–99, 112–113, 119, 121
Finkelhor, D., 18, 60
Finlay, T. J., 131
Fisch, R., 16, 36
Fishman, C., 32
Fleming, J., 95, 102
Flitcraft, A., 104
Flynn, J. P., 100
Ford, D. A., 104, 126–127
Forehand, R., 78, 85
Framo, J. L., 37
Frantz-Cook, A., 38, 47–54
Frazier, W., 104
Freeman, M. D. A., 95, 126, 132

Freud, S., 31, 94
Friedman, D. H., 68
Friedrich, W. N., 9
Friere, P., 159
Frieze, I. H., 104
Froland, C., 163
Fruchtman, L. A., 100, 105

G

Ganley, A. L., 11, 23, 38, 63–65, 140, 152
Garbarino, J., 140, 164
Garmezy, N., 81
Gayford, J. J., 97, 100
Geismar, L. C., 138–139
Gelinas, D. J., 13, 19
Geller, J. A., 32, 38
Gelles, R. J., 21, 58–61, 71, 93, 99–102, 105, 112–113, 137, 139, 141
George, V., 140, 142, 145
Giarretto, H., 18, 163
Giddings, W. C., 47, 49–51, 53–54
Gil, D., 44
Giles-Sims, J., 47–48, 50, 93, 95–96, 98, 101–102, 106–107, 122
Gilliam, G., 140
Gilligan, C., 15
Goldberg, D. P., 83
Goldner, V., 36, 144
Gondolf, E.W., 12, 18, 23, 38–39, 44, 57–58, 63, 68–69, 71, 113, 117, 134, 139, 141–142
Goode, W., 101
Gordon, D., 79
Gordon, L., 141
Gordon, R. C., 163
Greenspan, M., 30, 42–44, 162
Groth, A. N., 26
Grunebaum, H., 37
Grusznski, R., 69

H

Hackman, R. J., 157
Hammen, C., 79
Hall-McCorquodale, I., 16, 23

Hampton, K. L., 75
Hanks, S. E., 49
Hanneken, J., 63
Hansen, K. V., 60
Hanusa, D. R., 68
Hare-Mustin, R. T., 144
Hazlewood, L. R., 112–113, 117
Head, W. A., 158
Hendricks, D. R., 104
Hendricks, J., 104
Hershorn, M., 76, 84–85
Hess, R. D., 77
Hetherington, E. M., 76–77
Hill, M. H., 70
Hillier, V. F., 83
Hiroto, D., 79
Hofeller, K. H., 104
Hoffman, L., 101
Holmes, S. A., 130
Homant, R. J., 126, 133
Hughes, H. M., 76
Hughes, J. M., 75
Hymel, S., 82

I,J

Iannotti, R. J., 78
Jackson, D. D., 36
Jackson, D. N., 70
Jacobson, H. E., 119–121
Jaenicke, C., 79
Jaffe, P., 18, 24, 76–77, 79–80, 83, 85, 88, 104, 125–126, 128, 131, 133, 152, 154
Jaggar, A. M., 142–143
James, K., 140
Janes, C., 78
Jennings, J. L., 38–39
Johnson, J. M., 93, 96, 98–99, 112–113
Johnson, V. E., 13
Jouriles, E. N., 76
Joyce, S., 78, 85

K

Kanner, L., 31
Katcher, A., 31

Kates, M., 88
Katz, S., 152, 154
Kaufman, J., 80–81, 83
Kelly, J. B., 77
Kendall, P. C., 81
Kendall, S., 120
Kennedy, D. B., 126, 133
Kimboko, P., 163
Kincaid, P. J., 91
Kleckner, J., 140
Knoble, J., 104
Knowles, M., 131, 140
Kraft, S. P., 76, 78, 85
Kuhl, A. F., 102–103

L

Langley, R., 32, 93, 95–97, 102–103
LaPrairie, C., 118
Lauer, R. M., 83
Lawler, E. E. III, 157
Lebeaux, C. N., 140, 142, 145
LeClaire, D., 127–129, 133
Lerette, P., 130
Levens, B. R., 129
Levens, R. R., 104
Levy, R. C., 32, 93, 95–97, 102–103
Libow, J., 144–145
Lieber, L. L., 163
Lieberknecht, K., 98
Lion, J., 140
Long, N., 85
Lorion, R. P., 138–139
Loseke, D. R., 94, 103, 105–106, 119, 121, 127
Loving, N., 130
Lystad, M., 139

M

MacKinnon, L. K., 47
MacLeod, L., 21, 57–58, 93, 96, 98, 100–101, 103, 105, 109, 111, 116–119, 120, 134, 137, 152, 154–155, 163
Magill, J., 38, 51
Maidment, S., 132

Margolin, G., 38, 49
Martin, D., 32, 37, 59, 93, 95–96, 98, 100, 102, 104, 113
Masson, J. M., 13
Masters, W. H., 13
Maurer, L., 104–105, 122
Mayers, R., 65, 69
McCafferty, M., 160
McCall, G. J., 159, 163
McCormick, A. J., 21
McDonald, L., 93, 95–96, 98, 100, 102, 106–107, 114, 119–122
McEvoy, J. III, 142
McFall, R. M., 82
McIntosh, J., 119–121
McIntyre, D., 140
McKnight, J., 159
McLaughlin, A., 118
Meade-Ramrattan, J., 31
Meagher, M. S., 104
Micklow, P. L., 100
Middleton, B., 131
Miller, D., 47
Miller, J. B., 14, 43
Minuchin, S., 32, 36, 42, 47, 51, 140
Moore, D., 95–96, 125
Morash, M., 127
Mosk, M., 76
Muir, J., 127–129, 133
Myers, C., 68

N

Nadler, D. A., 157
Nairne, K., 30–31, 36, 42
Neidig, P. H., 68
Newton, P. J., 98, 102, 104, 107, 118, 122
Nichols, M. P., 37
Nickle, N., 38, 63–64

O,P

O'Brien, J., 101
Offord, D. R., 70
O'Leary, K. D., 13, 22, 24, 36, 76, 93, 96–97, 100

Pagelow, M. D., 59, 93, 95–96, 100, 102–105, 121
Pahl, J., 93–94, 96–98, 101–104, 106–107, 121, 126, 139
Painter, S. L., 96, 98
Pancoast, D., 163
Parkinson, G. C., 130
Penfold, P. S., 14, 42–44
Pepler, D., 88
Peressini, T., 93, 95–96, 98, 100, 102, 106–107, 114, 119, 120–122
Perry, D. G., 81
Perry, L. C., 81
Piven, F. F., 159
Pizzey, E., 95, 103–104, 111–112
Pollock, C. B., 9
Porter, C., 98
Porto, M. L., 31
Pressman, B., 16, 22–23, 25–26, 32, 36–37, 41, 44, 61, 63–67, 125, 134, 140, 142, 162
Purdy, F., 38, 63–64

R

Rappaport, J., 159
Raskin, P., 144–145
Rasmussen, P., 81
Rawlings, E. I., 42, 44
Rice, J., 104
Rickard, K. M., 78
Ridington, J., 95, 102, 112–114, 119, 121
Roberts, A. R., 59, 65, 120
Roberts, H., 158
Robey, A., 94, 140
Rohrbaugh, J. B., 44
Rosenbaum, A., 13, 22, 24, 36, 76, 84–85, 93, 96–97, 100
Rosenbaum, C. P., 49
Rosenberg, M. S., 78
Rosenwald, R. J., 94, 140
Rosewater, L. B., 97
Rothery, M., 163
Rounsaville, B. J., 95–97, 101–103, 105
Roy, M., 13, 22, 36, 95, 101–102, 125, 127
Rubin, K., 82
Russell, D., 12, 18, 38, 39, 44, 134

Rutter, M., 78–81, 84–85
Ryan, W., 158

S

Sample Survey and Data Bank Unit, 93, 98, 102–103, 106–107, 119, 120–122
Saunders, D. G., 38, 68
Schechter, S., 100–101, 111–113
Scheer, N. S., 93, 122
Schultz, L. G., 140
Schwartz, R., 37
Seligman, M. E. P., 98, 141
Shaevitz, M. H., 140
Shainess, N., 94, 140
Shapiro, C. H., 109
Shaw, D., 78, 85
Sherman, L. W., 104, 107, 128, 152, 154
Shumaker, S. A., 63
Shupe, A., 69, 112–113, 117
Siegel, S., 138
Simmons, J. L., 159, 163
Sinclair, D., 63–64, 134
Sines, J. O., 83
Skoretz, A., 164
Small, S. E., 16
Smillie, T., 93, 95–96, 98, 100, 102, 106–107, 114, 119–122
Smith, D. E., 13, 40
Smith, G., 30, 31, 36, 42
Smith, M. D., 98, 107
Snell, J. E., 94, 140
Snider, G., 164
Snyder, D. K., 93, 100, 105, 122
Sopp-Gilson, S., 24
Stacey, W. A., 69, 112–113, 117
Star, B., 32, 37–38, 63, 95, 97
Stark, E., 104
Stark, R., 142
Steele, B. F., 9
Steinfeld, G., 63
Steinmetz, S. K., 21, 58–61, 71, 101, 137, 141
Stewart, D. A., 60
Stone, L. H., 93, 105
Straus, M. A., 21, 58–61, 71, 101, 112–113, 137, 139, 141

Studer, M., 111–116
Sullivan-Hanson, J., 76, 85
Sutton, J., 141

T

Taggart, M., 54
Taub, N., 132
Taylor, J. W., 38, 47, 50, 54
Telford, A., 128, 133, 152, 154
Thorman, G., 127
Tierney, K. J., 111–113
Tomes, N., 141
Treger, H., 130
Trimble, D., 23
Truninger, E., 95, 104
Turner, S. F., 109

U,V

Urbain, E. S., 81
Ursel, E. J., 104, 132
Videka-Sherman, L., 163

W

Wahler, R. G., 163
Waites, E. A., 94–95
Walker, G. A., 14, 42–44

Walker, L. E., 37, 59, 61, 93, 95–100, 102,
    105, 139, 141
Wallerstein, J. S., 77
Washburn, 104
Wasserstrom, J., 38
Watzlawick, P., 16, 36
Weakland, J., 16, 36, 38
Weisstein, N., 31
Weitzman, J., 49–51, 53
Werk, A., 38, 51
Whittaker, J., 163
Wilde-Stevens, M., 118
Wilden, A., 54
Wilding, P., 140, 142, 145
Wilensky, H. L., 140, 142, 145
Wills, T. A., 163
Wilson, S. K., 24, 76–77, 79–80, 83, 85, 88,
Wintemute, M. J., 119–121
Withorn, A., 159
Wolfe, D. A., 24, 76–77, 79–80, 83, 85, 88,
    128, 131, 133, 152, 154
Wyckoff, H., 42–43
Wyman, E., 96
Wynn, M., 119

Z

Zahn-Waxler, C., 78
Zak, L., 24, 76–77, 79, 83, 85
Zigler, E., 80–81, 83
Zomnir, G., 104

Subject Index

A

Abused women
  characteristics of, 23-24,40,78,95-97
  empowerment of, see Empowerment,
    of women
  parentification and, 13
  professional helpers and, 8,104-105
  service delivery models for, 146-
    152,155-156
  shelters for, see Shelters for abused
    women
  social learning theory and, 100,141
  staying in assaultive relationships,
    6,13-14, 152
  because of economic dependence,
    99,102-103
  psychological explanations for, 94-
    100, 105-106
  sociological explanations for, 101-
    103, 105-106
  terminating assaultive relationships,
    93-110
  after termination, 106-108
  follow-up services for, 108-109
  therapeutic relationship with, 13-19
  treatment issues for, 26-27,45
  victimization and, 2,15,97-99
  See also Wife abuse; Women, violence
    against

Abusing men
  characteristics of, 13,22-23,32,45,59
  criminal charging of, 132-133,155
  theories for behavior of, 59-62
  treatment of, 62-72
    court-mandated,65-66,71-72,152,154
    effectiveness of, 68-69
    group counseling in, 38-39,63-64,139
    integrated approach to, 61-62
    issues in, 28-29
    programs for, 58,62,63-64,137-
      138,141
    research on, problems of, 71-72
Adler, Alfred, 3
Alcohol, as factor in wife abuse, 11,140
Anger management programs, 12,139
Assaultive husbands, see Abusing men
Attitudes Towards Women Scales, 96-97

B

Basic Personality Inventory, 70
Battered women, see Abused women
BEM Sex-Role Inventory, 97

C

Chicoutimi Follow-Up Program, 108
Child sexual abuse, 13,18,26

Children
    effects of family violence on, 5-
        6,22,24-25,61-62,75-91
        research on, 76-86
        treatment issues for, 27-28
    as factor in family violence, 59
    parentification and, 13,25
    primary prevention programs for, 91
    sex role socialization of, 61-62
    in shelters for abused women, 86-
        90,108,120,154
Chiswick's Women's Aid, 112
Circular causality, in family systems
    therapy, 4,35-36,49-50,144
Clergy, as helpers of abused women, 104
Community development, principles of,
    158-159
Couple therapy, 38,45
Criminal justice system, see Legal sys-
    tem
Crisis intervention
    for children in shelters, 89-90
    as secondary prevention, 138-139
Cycle of violence, 81,98-99,154

D

Deutsch, Helene, 31
Discovery House (Calgary), 108

E

Earlscourt Child and Family Centre,
    Reception Classroom, 77,79,88-89
Empowerment
    community development perspective
        of, 161-162
    of women, 2,6,128,133
        as therapeutic goal, 2,8,12,43,52

F

Family Assessment Device, 70
Family Conflict Tactics Scale, 122

Family Consultant Service (London,
    Ont.), 131
Family Services of Winnipeg, 108
Family systems therapy
    and legal protectionist shelters, 115-
        116
    in treatment of wife abuse, 4,47-
        55,144-145
    criticism of, 16-17,32-37,47,50,54
    intervention models, 50-55
    theory of, 49-51,101-102
Family Trouble Clinic (Detroit), 130
Feminist therapy
    social work students' attitudes
        toward, 160
    in treatment of wife abuse, 3-4,16,42-
        45,49, 144-145,162
    theory of, 60-61,142-143
Feminists
    opposition to wife abuse, 2,113
    shelters for abused women and, 111-
        113,114-115
    types of, 143
Freud, Sigmund, 3,13,31,94

G

General Health Questionnaire, 83
Greater Montreal Social Services Centre,
    108
Group treatment, 38-42,44
    for abusing men, 5,63-64,68,69
    psychoeducational focus of, 38-39
    closed groups in, case for, 41
    leadership issue in, 39-40,64-65,67-68

H

Hamilton-Wentworth Family Violence
    Treatment Program, 63,66-67
    evaluation of, 69-71
Helpers, see Professional helpers
Home Environment Questionnaire, 83
Huron Street School Reception Class-
    room, 89

J

Jung, Carl, 3
Justice system, *see* Legal system

L

Lawyers, as helpers of abused women,
104
Leadership
in group counseling, 39-40
with assaultive husbands, 64-65,67-
68
Legal system
abusing men and, 65-66,132-133,155
child sexual abuse and, 18
wife abuse and, 7,9-10,17-18,142
Lincoln County Board of Education,
primary prevention programs of,
91
London Battered Women's Advocacy
Clinic, 96,97,108

M

Masochism, female, 13,94-95
Melfort Safe Homes, 108
Mental illness, abused women and,
97,140
Minneapolis Domestic Violence Experi-
ment, 128
Minnesota Multiphasic Personality In-
ventory, 97
Minuchin, Salvador, family systems
therapy and, 32-35,36-37,51,53,140

N

National Clearinghouse on Family
Violence, 116
Nellie's Second Stage House (Toronto),
108
Neutrality, in family systems therapy,
36-37

P

Parentification, 13,25
Perry Self-Efficacy Scale, 81,82
Philadelphia Child Guidance Center, 32
Police
charging of abusing men, 125-
126,128-129,132-133,152,154,155
social service activities of, 129-131
wife abuse and, 7,104,125,126-131
Power
in feminist theory, 60,61,142,143
social structure of, 2,9,12
Primary prevention, 138-139
programs of, for children, 91
Professional helpers, wife abuse and,
8,104-105, 113,162,164
Psychologists, treatment of wife abuse
and, 104
Psychotherapy, criticism of, 2-3,13,29-
32,42

R

RAVEN, abusing men's program, 141
Rehabilitation, as tertiary prevention,
138
Royal Commission on the Status of
Women, 11

S

Secondary prevention, 138-139
for children in violent families, 90
Shelters for abused women, 6-7,84-
85,104,111-123
in Canada, 57,87,111-113,116-
121,137,152
effects of
on terminating assaultive relationships, 105
on violence reduction, 122-123
feminists and, 111-113, 114-115
follow-up programs in, 108-109,120
government support and, 113-114,
117

intervention programs for children in, 86-90
professional helpers and, 113,164
types of, 114-116
use of, 154
women's needs and, 118-120
Social Information Problem Solving Interview, 82
Social learning theory
abused women and, 100,141
abusing men and, 4-5,61-62,64,141
children and, 80
Social workers, treatment of wife abuse and, 104

T

Television, gender role stereotyping and, 11
Tertiary prevention, 138
Therapists
advocacy/protection roles of, 18
biases of, 23-24,162
treatment of abused women and, 13-19
Transition House (Vancouver), 112
Transition houses, *see* Shelters for abused women

V

Victimization, 2,15,48,97-99
Violent families, characteristics of, 25-26, 79-80

W

Walker Cycle Theory of Violence, 98-99

Wife abuse
causation theories of, 139-146
preventive strategies based on, 146-152
community development perspective on, 157-165
community norms and, 9-10,127
definition of, 134
legal sanctions against, 17-18, 132-133,155
non-physical forms of, 21, 22, 31, 39,137
prevention of, 137-156
integrated approach to, 143-146
service model for, 155-156
psychoanalytic view of, 13,29-32,42-43
psychological theories on, 94-100,140-141
sociocultural theories on, 141-143
statistics on, 57-58,125,137
See also Abused women; Women, violence against
Women
discrimination against, 10-12
empowerment of, *see* Empowerment, of women
Freudian concepts of, 3,13,31
sex role socialization of, 17,133, 142
social norms and, 14-15,17,22,23
violence against
cultural norms and, 1-2,21,42,44,141-142
as focus of feminist therapy, 39,45,49-50,60
power and, 2,6,12
See also Abused women; Wife abuse
Women in Second Stage (Winnipeg), 108

For Product Safety Concerns and Information please contact our EU
representative GPSR@taylorandfrancis.com Taylor & Francis Verlag GmbH,
Kaufingerstraße 24, 80331 München, Germany

Printed and bound by CPI Group (UK) Ltd, Croydon, CR0 4YY
08/06/2025
01896998-0012